T0171615

OR EYES

How to avoid a trip to the OR

Kathleen E. Volpe-Schaffer RN

iUniverse, Inc.
Bloomington

OR Eyes
How to avoid a trip to the OR

Copyright © 2012 Kathleen E. Volpe-Schaffer RN

iUniverse books may be ordered through booksellers or by contacting:

iUniverse
1663 Liberty Drive
Bloomington, IN 47403
www.iuniverse.com
1-800-Authors (1-800-288-4677)

ISBN: 978-1-4502-5049-8 (sc)
ISBN: 978-1-4502-5050-4 (e)

Printed in the United States of America

iUniverse rev. date: 6/7/2012

Introduction

We can all agree that being sick is not a pleasant experience. Needing an operation and going to the operating room is an even less joyous occasion. Everyone has a story to tell of their operation. Some are scary and some are funny, and some are just plain weird. Being nervous about being a patient in the OR is expected. You wouldn't be normal if you weren't a little on edge. But don't worry, because the outcomes are almost always good. I've scrubbed and or circulated for hundreds, if not thousands of surgical procedures over my operating room nurse's career and I have never ceased to be surprised and amazed with each experience. Over the last three decades many operative procedures have been altered, modified, shortened and tweaked in order to provide better patient outcomes. Hospital stays are shorter, despite being more expensive, but that's another topic. Patients are happier about shorter hospital stays. It used to be, say in the 1970s that if you were diagnosed with breast cancer, regardless how small the mass, your only option was to have a mastectomy, the total removal of your breast. Today lumpectomy, the removal of only the tumor and some surrounding tissue

1

is the choice of many women and long term prognosis has improved despite less invasive procedures. Today, often times it is undetectable to anyone that you had any breast surgery at all, provided you're not standing there naked. But hospital operating rooms are busier than ever. We keep doing the same procedures over and over. The baby boomer bulge of the population, those born post WWII from 1945 to 1965 is aging and obesity and Diabetes are on the rise exponentially, as well as the surgical procedures needed to allay the effects of these conditions. Even though surgical procedures and methods have changed over the decades, the patients' stories and the reasons why they are visiting the operating room have not. These medical conditions and the stories that precluded their visits to the OR have moved me in such a way that I have no excuse not to share them with you, primarily for the sake of education and disease prevention. I've seen too many scenarios that could have turned out differently if only the disease, the cancer, the diabetes, or the lump was caught earlier, or if only someone told them what to look for. My goal is to inform people on how to take control of their lifestyles by recognizing the risks of disease development and thereby avoiding that dreaded trip to the Operating Room. All of the patients I talk about have a story to tell and they speak to the major health issues that impact our society today, just as strongly as they did 30 years ago. These diseases and conditions are still as controversial as they were 30 years ago. AIDS, abortion, breast cancer, obesity (on the rise), diabetes (on the rise too), and organ donation are just a few scenarios explored. The sad story is that even though great strides have been made in the early detection and treatments of these conditions, their numbers are not really dwindling. The real horror story is that the incidences of these conditions are increasing. So I asked myself, "Why?"

The Nursing profession is responsible for many actions related to health care but probably one of the most import functions of nursing is disease prevention via health education. So I've decided to take a different approach; I can teach others what I've seen and know though my experiences as an OR nurse; to teach from my nursing perspective, to teach from a personal point of view from inside my patients' bodies as they lay on the OR table, and not as a text book set of rules because these are real people. I want you to know these people personally, exactly like I did and maybe the impact will be more empowering. Many people think "Oh, that only happens to other people, not me." And some people will make up some home made reasoning as to why that condition doesn't apply to them. "I'm too tall" or "That only happens to that group of people", or the best excuse and state of denial is the line "That doesn't run in my family!"

Yea, right! Life is full of twists and turns and decisions must me made and sometimes we incorrectly or unknowingly take the rocky path. That is the goal of this book; to empower people to choose that right, that smoother road and to make those easier and better decisions toward the goal of optimal health. One of the best things we can do is to learn from our errors, our mistakes. But an easier and less painful route to take is to learn how to not repeat the follies of others. I call these "Other Peoples' Mistakes" or OPMs; for example, smoking. I've come across a plethora of these incorrect life choices impacting life's outcomes and I wish to share them with you in order to empower you. We are all potential OR patients and we need to be armed with the best possible information so you too can avoid that trip to the OR. Take it from me, I've seen the worst of the worst in the OR.

I've compiled various surgical scenarios from my nursing and operating room experiences, taking an almost historical perspective and incorporating different yet common diseases that I've seen firsthand, on the OR table and have witnessed through my "OR EYES" and participated in surgically treating. Examples are procedures treating the consequences of diabetes and breast cancer, lung cancer, drunk driving and organ donation, abortion, and drug abuse just to name a few. My hope is that this book can be a learning experience for anyone who reads it, without having to experience it. I have witnessed the most distressing worst case scenarios through these "OR EYES". A few are absolutely disgusting. Some have a funny side, but many in my opinion are horribly tragic and I would have not believed it if I didn't see it for myself with my own "OR EYES." The saddest thing is that in most of the diseases referenced here, all were and are preventable conditions or at least easily managed if detected early. Hopefully this book will help to provide awareness of preventative pro-active solutions that can easily be incorporated into your everyday activities which will prove to provide wellness and longevity. We're all OR patients sooner or later, but hopefully later; correction- or hopefully never!

CHAPTER 1

FED UP

I couldn't take it anymore. I needed a change. My only question was whether or not I could handle all the blood, guts, pus and other oozing types of drainage the job would entail. But I finally did it. I couldn't believe that I landed a job in an operating room. I nervously applied to a major inner city university hospital operating room and was hired immediately as full time R.N. I was especially surprised that I was hired without any operating room experience. "They must be desperate", I thought to myself. There was always a shortage of nurses as far back in time as I could remember. I knew it was a done deal as soon as I flashed my state of Pennsylvania professional RN license in front of the recruiting head nurse's bulging eyes as she snatched it from my hands. Val, the OR manager said to me with a big simile on her face, "We'll just keep this on file and display it in the nursing administrative office for legal and safe keeping reasons". That made sense to me, because I knew that all licensed professionals, nurses, doctors, physical therapists, social workers and alike must have their current licenses on file in the Human Resources departments, as it is a federal and state law. It is mandated by the Joint Commission on the Credentialing of Hospitals. This is a federal agency that oversees that the people you hire are really the people you hire, and that the person wielding the license is a state tested and professionally qualified individual. All professional licenses are color marked and printed on special paper to cut down on counterfeiting, just like money.

I went to work in the operating room because I was wiped out from my previous job as a surgical intensive care unit (SICU) nurse. Working in the SICU was an exhausting endeavor. Rotating shift work was wicked. I was working swing shifts from 11pm to 7am, and then jumping to 3pm to 11pm eight hours later in the very same day. I rarely worked the 7 am to 3 pm shift. It seemed like I was always low man on the totem pole. I was always paying my dues. But what made this so difficult was the fact that I always had to be as sharp as a tack because this SICU job required specialized and highly technically demanding skills, and there is no room for error. Running codes, watching EKG monitors, interpreting arrhythmias, taking vital signs, doing dressing changes, assessing urine out and fluids taken, and calculating IV drips, along with attending to your tracheotomy patient on the noisy ventilator were routine daily tasks.

Taking care of intubated respirator dependent patients was just a mega responsibility that demanded my most constant attention. God forbid if I rubbed my tired eyes or blinked at the wrong moment. One specific intubated patient will forever taint my memory. A twenty four hour fresh post-op open heart surgery CABG patient finally woke up. He had just regained enough consciousness to realize where he was and proceeded to just yank out his endotracheal tube (ET) from his throat and trachea. He did a good job except he did it when no one was watching. The tape securing the ET in place on his face kept it from being completely removed. So what happened next, he began to choke and vomit and he aspirated the vomitus from his throat and mouth back into his lungs. But he couldn't clear his mouth because half of the ET was still in his mouth and partially in his throat, stimulating his gag reflex. He was vomiting violently. This was a bad sign because he was now attempting to breath in his vomitus with nowhere to go except back into his lungs. He had no control of his airway because of his misplaced ET. It was bad again because even though he had no food in his stomach, his gut was still producing the hydrochloric acid (HCL) needed for food digestion and the anesthetics used in surgery to decrease secretions had worn off. Hydrochloric acid in the lungs can be fatal. Digestion of lung tissue is a death sentence. It burns and damages and then scars the lung tissue which renders them unable to do their life sustaining job; breathing. The main culprit of HCL in the lungs is what is known as the development of "aspiration pneumonia." The Ph. of stomach acid-HCl, is approximately 2.5, which is very acidic and it can be compared to inhaling bleach. Aspiration pneumonia is a chemical burn of the trachea, bronchus and the little alveoli sacs of the lungs. Aspiration pneumonia is the most lethal form of pneumonia. Up to thirty (30%) to fifty (50 %) of patients with aspiration pneumonia will die because of it, and or develop lifelong consequences due to its incidence.

Unfortunately, this patient did develop aspiration pneumonia and died a week later. His open heart surgery was a success, but he died because of a complication. His death became a morbidity statistic. Prevention of aspiration pneumonia is the main reason surgery patients are instructed to stop eating foods and drinking liquids 8 hours before receiving general anesthesia. After this unfortunate incident, we started partially restraining post operative patient's hands, just enough so they could not reach their mouths and remove their endotracheal tubes.

Besides these ventilator dependent patients, just taking care of a patient's individual needs, the turning and lifting of people who were two to three times my weight, and doing all of this for 2 or 3 patients at a time paved my way to the exit. I just couldn't do it anymore. Of course the SICU where I worked was always short staffed; someone was always calling out sick. I learned early on that it was the norm in the nursing profession to work with a skeleton crew. There was always a nurse who was left over from the previous shift who was doing some form of limited mandatory overtime. Nurses quit as rapidly as they were hired.

I quickly discovered that working in a specialty unit like the operating room insured me less weekend duty as well as less rotation to holidays and to the evening and night shifts as well. Weekend rotation in the OR was only once every 6 weeks vs. every other as in the SICU. "I could handle this" I thought to myself. This is because in the OR, 99% of all the surgeries are elective and are performed on the weekdays. It was more or less a controlled schedule. After all, surgeons don't like working nights or weekends either. Weekends and nights in the

OR were minimally staffed. Only emergency cases like appendectomies, organ transplants, or trauma cases were penciled onto the schedule after 3 pm. So in essence, we OR nurses followed the doctors' schedules. I liked that.

While working in the SICU I realized that my internal clock was whacked and severely skewed to the left. Sleeping 3 to 4 hours a day for three or four straight days, I found was not conducive to optimal health. I ate my meals on the run and I lost weight. I was six pounds lighter than what I was 6 months prior. Sleep deprivation made me feel sick in a weird way. I felt that my brain was atrophying. Lack of sleep is extremely taxing on one's body. I didn't start drinking coffee until I became a nurse. Caffeine was a necessary addiction, despite coffee's bitter taste. But I discovered that I could fix that problem. I doused each cup of coffee with at least three heaping teaspoons of sugar and the more cream the better. Out of necessity, I think I invented the coffee milkshake back in 1976.

I realized I needed more normalcies in my life. I was consistently absent from family functions because of working crazy swing shifts. Christmas was just another day on my calendar when I would earn time and a half and be even more exhausted because everyone else in the SICU got off and I was doing twice as much work. I needed an out. I was frying myself to a crisp.

I looked weekly in the Sunday Philadelphia Inquirer newspaper scanning the nursing jobs, hoping to pinpoint a possible job interview. I needed so desperately to escape the stress of this SICU job. The year was 1977. Two weeks into my search I zeroed in on a position as a cardiac catheterization nurse at another University hospital.

Despite the location of the University, I eagerly dialed the phone number. My interview with a cardiologist was scheduled for the following Friday. When the day of my interview arrived, I was pumped! I made sure that everything was perfect. I tweaked my resume to perfection. Being a veteran SICU nurse I knew that I was more than qualified. I even bought a new suit for the interview. I was optimistic.

I arrived a half hour early at 10:00am for my 10:30am appointment. I sat in the waiting room tapping my feet to the faint barely audible Frank Sinatra tune. Promptly at 10:30, I was ushered into the doctor's office. I sat again, waiting patiently. When Dr. P entered, we exchanged the usual self intros and the interview began. He asked the usual questions like where I went to school and how long I worked in critical care. I thought I was doing just fine. Just when I thought he was going to offer me the job, the most unexpected thing happened. Dr. P leaned forward and with a stern look on his face, he said to me, "I'm sorry Kathy. You are not what I'm looking for to fill the position."

"I don't understand", I replied.

"Let me explain. I think you are more than qualified for the job, but it's your age."

I thought to myself, "What does my age have to do with anything?" So I asked him, "So, why should that matter?"

I was 22 years old at the time.

His reply angered me. "What if you get pregnant?" he asked me.

"But I'm not married", I snapped back at him. "And besides, what does my fertility have to do with anything?" I was furious and humiliated at the same time. I couldn't believe that a stranger, a man, a supposedly PROFESSIONAL, would have the gall to ask such a personal, intimate question, and especially of another professional. I immediately realized that his preconceived attitude was the problem; he didn't see me as a professional. He was judging me because I was a woman, a woman of childbearing age, and not on my abilities to perform the job. But most disturbing to me was the fact that he posed that degrading question to a younger woman, who was obviously in a dependent, subservient role. In retrospect, when I think back to that time, almost 30 years ago, I realize now that I was a victim of sexual discrimination. I wasn't seen as an equal professional because I was female. I thought to myself, "What if I was a man applying for this job? Would this doc not hire a male applicant if he and his wife were thinking about becoming pregnant? And would he have the nerve to ask another man about his fertility prospects?" I believed that I didn't get the job because I was a YOUNG FEMALE, with the potential to become pregnant! I was being unfairly judged because of my gender, and age, and fertility status. I believe my personal life was none of his business. Most importantly, he made me feel dirty and unworthy. I sensed that my future and my career choices were being manipulated by this man in an authoritative position, and who had control over me because I was female. The fact that he didn't hire me because he thought I would become pregnant is even more disgusting. I was actually embarrassed. I felt so disrespected. But I refused to be humiliated by this jerk. I couldn't wait to leave his office. I realized at that moment that I didn't want his 9 to 5 job anyway. I'd rather have nothing than have his job. I thanked MR. P. for his consideration for the job interview and promptly left. I turned the table on him. He was just another sanctimonious jerk in my eyes. I felt terribly hurt after that interview.

So I quit the SICU without a new job, or a paycheck on the horizon. Two weeks later I was hired for the OR at Thomas Jefferson University Hospital. Thankfully the hiring process at Jeff was a breeze and nothing like my last demeaning encounter. At last I found my dream job as an operating room nurse; an OR nurse. But most importantly, I would be working daylight hours 7am to 3:30pm. I found that working daylight shifts, like the 7am to 3pm or 10am to 6:30pm, Mondays through Fridays was my dream job come true! But what I did not expect from my new employment at Jeff was indeed the most valuable aspects of my 30 plus year nursing career, as well as in my life. I encountered the desperation of souls to become well again, and the human spirit that dwells within to thrive despite the odds, all through the vision of my OR Eyes. I witnessed the intensity of both the physical human pain, along with its mental anguish. What I learned and saw in the operating room cannot be taught in any text books. I worked there for over 10 years and I saw it all; it consumed me.

CHAPTER 2

THE UROLOGY SUITE

After rotating through the various operative specialties, I chose to work in the Urology division of the operating room. The cases were diverse and the pace moved quickly. Everything was a snap. Urology is the branch of medical science dealing with the urinary or urogenital tracts and its disorders. From the tip of the penis to the kidney, if it needed surgery I was involved. I assisted in hundreds of transurethral resections of the prostate (TURPs) and transurethral resections of bladder tumors (TURBTs), prostate biopsies, and bladder biopsies in both men and women. As any middle aged and senior man knows, enlargement of prostate gland is as ubiquitous as gray hair in this age group. As a man ages, his prostate gland just naturally enlarges. The enlargement is benign in and of itself, but when it becomes large enough to compress on a man's urethra he'll display urinary symptoms. There are medicines today in the 21st century that have demonstrated some success with shrinking the prostate and alleviating those bothersome symptoms, but back in the 1970's there were none. Having a TURP was the more common route. Inserting a stainless steel rod the size of a milk shake straw, that can accommodate a cauterizing (burning) loop on the tip, 12 inches into a man's penis is/ was the typical procedure. Having an enlarged prostate is especially bothersome at nighttime. When it gets to the point where a man cannot pee at all, often times is when he'll finally call the doctor. Needless to say, most of my day in the urological suite of the OR was spent caring for these gentlemen undergoing a TURP. It was typically a quick and painless procedure thanks to epidural anesthesia. These procedures took less than an hour and it was not unusual that we could do ten of them within an eight hour time span. I assisted the team of urologists everyday in every aspect of surgical intervention on the urinary tract, ranging from cases as critical as kidney transplants to the benign and uneventful vasectomy.

Then one day the most unusual case entered the URO suite. On this particular afternoon while I was working the lunch break shift, 10am to 6pm, the urologist working the Uro suite that day told me that he had an emergency he had to plug into the schedule immediately. He told me he had to cancel the remaining three TURPs for the day, and to prepare the OR suite for a general laparotomy (abdominal surgery) procedure. "What kind of lap will we be doing?" I asked. "What are you looking for?"

The urologist replied, "It's really not going to be a laparotomy. I just want to have a general abdominal surgical instrument tray handy, just in case." He really didn't answer my question so I really didn't know what to expect. A general laparotomy tray held a larger array of instruments, like forceps, hemostats, scissors and retractors.

"And oh yea, have a bunch of 20cc to 50cc syringes with large bore 18ga needles on hand", the surgeon said to me as he exited the room. I couldn't imagine why in the world he would need those things either. I didn't ask, and besides he left the suite too fast. In retrospect, I should have.

Needless to say, when the present case finished we turned the room around in 10 minutes. "Turning the room around" meant terminally cleaning it. Every piece of furniture, the bed, the desks, any blood soiled articles, and sometimes the walls got bloody too, were wiped down with a disinfectant. Ten minutes later the door to my OR room slammed open. Our next "victim" was being wheeled into the OR suite by a young and very strong nursing assistant named Vince. "Vinny", as all the nurses lovingly called him was our senior nursing assistant. He had a movie star smile and always a sparkle in his eye. Everybody loved Vinny. He was kind, funny, and always the perfect gentleman, but more importantly he could safely lift the heaviest, and or the most morbidly obese patient and correctly place the patient into whatever position that was needed for any surgical procedure. Vinny was hard working, and we all needed him. He was a valuable asset to our OR. We, the nurses had to share him between the 8 operating rooms on our floor. If he wasn't running specimens to the path lab, he was picking up patients from their rooms. Vinny was the nicest person you could ever know. But Vinny was off limits to our female fantasies, primarily because work romances were scorned upon, and unfortunately but more importantly Vinny was gay! And he was proud of it, as anyone should be, regardless of anyone's sexual orientation. This concept was a first for me. Now, bear in mind, this was 1978. Just to know Vinny, he unwittingly taught everyone the most valuable attribute a person could demonstrate; Diversity. Every person deserves respect. We human beings are all created equal, and the proof lies in the fact that when the gunshot victim who is exsanguinating to death on the OR table needs multiple units of blood in order to save his life, that precious liquid is donated and administered without prejudice as to the donor's race, color, religious beliefs, nationality, sexual orientation, age, language spoken, or gender. So if anyone should have an ego problem regarding their biases, you need to get over yourself, and realize that you are no better than anyone else, because of all of the millions of gallons of human blood I've probably ever seen, washed my hands of, smelled, measured, wiped up, slipped on, touched, and hung while working in the OR, it all looked exactly the same to me! When someone is bleeding to death in the OR from a MVA, they don't question the donor's race, religion or ethnicity, just as long as they wake up. Vinny was everybody's friend, and everyone loved him. He was a team player and he was the best, and no one gave a crap about his sexual orientation. That's the way it should be, always.

The OR staff frequently and jokingly, but under our breaths so as not to let the patients hear us, referred to the patients as "victims." Perhaps this gesture was a way of alleviating the stress of our jobs. After all, who looks forward to going under the knife? I think we were relieved that it was happening to someone else and not ourselves, despite everyone knowing that surgery in this day and age is extremely safe. It is a hospital not "The House on Haunted Hill!" The door to OR suite #10 abruptly opened as Vinny wheeled in our next victim, our emergency case, through the doorway. The patient was a young black man who was fully awake, alert and oriented. He correctly identified himself as the person wearing the same name ID bracelet that was stapled onto his left wrist. For patient privacy identification purposes, I'll just call him John. John was my father's name. To tell you the truth I don't remember the patient's name. That's the first thing every OR nurse does before any surgical procedure is performed; correctly identify the patient. Many a disaster has been prevented by correctly identifying the patient, and then operating on the correct person and or the correct body part, but that's another chapter. John transported himself from the gurney to the OR bed with minimal assistance from Vinny. John did not seem to be in any distress. As a matter of fact, he seemed too comfortable. He answered my questions in a calm tone of voice. He smiled incessantly. To me this scenario seemed odd. I wondered what kind of emergent operation he needed to have done. John could not have been any older than thirty years old. He denied any allergies to any medicines or foods. He was very articulate and business like as well. I pulled up his hospital gown, just a little and placed a bovie plate on his right thigh. I next buckled the 6 inch wide safety belt snugly around and just above his knees. I quickly scanned the operative permit. The date noted on the consent was today's date. John's signature was present on the sign here XX line. The anesthesiologist then snatched the chart away from my grasp before I could look at the line which stated what kind of operative procedure was documented on the permit. One moment later, John's anesthetized body peacefully fell into slumber mode. The scrub nurse precisely arranged her back table and her field tray. We did our sponge, sharp, and hemostat counts and I placed the kick sponge buckets to within the scrub nurse's throwing range. Then I connected the bovie cord to the bovie cauterizing machine. The surgeons entered the room with hands and elbows dripping water from their 5 minute surgical hand scrub. They donned their sterile gowns and gloved, except for the resident who would prep the patient's surgical field. I approached from behind on my tippy toes and adjusted the overhead lamps, directing the high intensity beams of light down onto the patient's abdomen. I tuned on the radio station to the local news channel. Finally, I sat down and started reviewing the chart. To me, the patient's chart was like a book that helped pass the time. Many OR cases can be absolutely long and boring. But that is a good thing because everyone wants the operation to go smooth and uneventful. Frequently, I viewed reading a patient's chart as entertaining. I was always curious to know how patients presented their symptoms to their primary caregivers, and then what tests the doctor ordered and the kinds of diseases or conditions the doctor was ruling out. Finally, when the conclusion or the diagnosis was reached, I was relieved to see the mystery solved. To me every chart read like an Agatha Christi novel. Some more mysterious and complicated than others, but most were pretty obvious and straightforward.

John lay on the operative table unconscious and motionless from the initial round of anesthetic agents. His heartbeat could be heard and visualized on the cardiac monitor as a steady and regular 76 beats per minute. I could not see the operative field as clearly as the surgeons or scrub nurse, as I was a good 10 to 15 feet away. Frequently, as a circulating nurse, because you are not "sterile" the closest you can get to the operative field is about 2 to 3 feet. An example would be when the scrub nurse or one of the surgeons were to pass off the operative specimen. The senior 4th year urology resident, who was to prep John's surgical site, approached John and started to apply the betadine solution to John's lower abdomen, his genital area with the usual orange colored iodine solution. As I opened John's chart and started to read, I thought I heard one of the residents giggle. Simultaneously, as my vision focused to read the operative procedure John signed for, I immediately became very aware of what the giggling was in reference to. From my sitting stool I glanced over to the operative field. I wanted to die of embarrassment when I saw what I saw. I arose from my chair and walked closer to the sterile field,

Approximately six feet away from me, with the help of one of the residents, dancing circles in the air was John's edematous, definitely erect penis. With the help of the same 4th year resident "It" was pointing upward as erect as a California Redwood, staring straight at me. I dared not look. I looked back down to the chart and continued to read the operative permit. It stated, "Evacuation of priapism, penile venous blood". Was I embarrassed? No. Why should I be? It was work. Well, maybe just a little embarrassed. Being the only female in the room and outnumbered 4 men to 1 woman, I knew for sure that I better not giggle back. Thank goodness I was wearing the usual OR garb which included a face mask, so nobody could really see my facial gestures, at least not clearly. I couldn't laugh like the guys were, at least not out loud.

That would be unprofessional. Did the residents laugh and giggle on purpose in front of me? Probably.

I had only read about priapism in medical text books in nursing school, but I had never actually seen one. What a weird word "priapism" was. Later on I took the opportunity to research the condition. The word priapism originated from the Greek God "Priapus". Priapus was the Greek God of fertility. He was the son of Aphrodite, the Greek God of love. Priapus was known for his huge genitalia, hence the name of the condition "Priapism".

OK. I understood. But why did the doctors need those huge needles? The head surgeon and the residents used the large bore 18 gauge needles to puncture the veins in Johns swollen penis to relieve the engorged blood within them. The surgeons drained approximately 20cc of dark red blood from the tortuous vessels of John's penis. The operation took about a half an hour, at the most from start to finish. It was pretty quick. When John was taken to the recovery room, he was responsive, but still groggy from the anesthesia. His penis was wrapped with thick kling gauze. He also had a urinary catheter inserted into his penis to ensure an intact urine outflow. But most importantly, his penis was no longer rigid. Whether or not John would remain potent, only time would tell.

But why did John have priapism? I learned how Priapism is no laughing matter. It is truly a medical emergency. I wondered what could possibly cause such a freakish condition. I found the answer documented in John's chart. It all made so much sense to me. John's past medical history revealed that he was a cocaine addict, among other substance abuse addictions. John was a professional and he hid his illicit drug usage perfectly.

Rather than shoot up into his muscular biceps, like into his brachial veins, he would shoot up his cocaine into the vessels in his penis! OUCH !!! The chronic puncturing and subsequent scarring in the veins of his penis due to the numerous injections of a probably not too sterile concoction eventually corroded the once smooth and supple endothelial linings of the veins in John's penis. Adhesions and scar formations formed in his penile veins and these narrowed veins subsequently caused blockage of the normal blood flow from his penis. The narrowed lumens in the veins in his penis acted like bottle necks that prevented the blood from draining back into his circulatory system. He could not become flaccid. But the erection in priapism is a paradoxical erection. It is not the result of sexual stimulation as one might think it should be. Nor is it relieved by ejaculation. It's not that easy. John's erection was pathological or abnormal. It was also very painful, as is typical in cases of priapism.

I read in John's chart that his erection started 24 to 48 hours ago. As desirable as one might think this is, it is not at all a wanted condition. Time is of the essence when it comes to preserving a man's potency. The duration of the symptoms of priapism is critical to the outcome. A recent Scandinavian study reports that 92% of patients with priapism for less than 24 hours will remain potent. Conversely, only 22 % of patients with priapism that lasted longer than 7 days remained potent. So the longer priapism lasts, the worse the outlook for preserving a man's potency. Advice to all men: Just like the commercials on TV say, any erection lasting longer than 4 hours needs prompt urgent medical attention. The longer medical treatment is delayed, the greater the risk for permanent erectile dysfunction.

My research also revealed some important and interesting information about priapism. It is more common than you would think. Priapism of course, only affects men. It affects more Africans than any other race. John was African American. Priapism occurs in all age groups. But the most interesting risk factor in the development of priapism and its relation to the African population is that Sickle Cell trait is the #1 predisposing factor in the incidence of priapism. Leukemia and malaria are also risk factors. Sickle Cell anemia, as well as having the sickle cell trait is a genetic condition found primarily in the African population. This means that it is an inherited genetic condition. The abnormal curved or sickle shape of red blood cells clump together, forming little blood clots that block blood flow. I did not see this documented on John's chart if he had Sickle Cell Disease (SCD) or the trait. Maybe it wasn't documented. Or maybe the doctors didn't test for it. I don't know. But I wasn't looking for it either. However, any adult male using intracavernosal (indictable medicines into the penile shaft) agents and other medicines is the cause of approximately 21-80 % of priapism cases. This is what John did. He was injecting cocaine into the veins of his penis and that was the predisposing factor and/or the cause his priapism. In the western world, men using oral erectile dysfunction agents account for only 0.05 -6% of priapism cases. That's a very small amount. This latter group is more educated and seeks medical attention earlier. In all other cases, sickle cell trait is the leading cause. According to Pasrraga-Marquez (2004) the rate of priapism in adults with sickle cell disease (SCD) is as high as 89%. In children, approximately two thirds of pediatric patients who have priapism also have SCD (Parraga-Marquez, 2004).

In conclusion, there are many other diseases that can be associated with priapism, and the taking of certain medications also contributes to its incidence. All are beyond the scope of this book. Please consult with your primary care practitioner if you should experience penile erection for longer than four hours. I would not have believed it if I didn't see it for myself through my OR Eyes in the OR!

CHAPTER 3

SUGAR IS NOT ALWAYS SWEET

Let's talk about something that touches everyone's life. Everyone knows of, or is related to someone who has some form of diabetes mellitus (DM). Diabetes is not a disease that can be cured by any surgical procedure, but its devastating consequences are frequently and almost always treated surgically in the operating room. I swear, operating rooms and surgeons would not be as busy as they are if it weren't for diabetes. The word diabetes is of German origin. Its translation means "passing through". Mellitus is of German origin as well and the prefix "meli's" translation means "honey". Taber's medical dictionary defines "mellitus" as a disorder of carbohydrate metabolism, characterized by elevated levels of glucose (sugar) in the blood and urine resulting from inadequate production or utilization of the hormone insulin. We frequently see in DM how glucose (sugar) **"passes through"** the kidneys and can be detected readily in both one's urine as elevated acetone due to increased fat metabolism detected with a dip stick and as elevated glucose levels in blood testing. Normal blood levels of glucose (sugar) should range between 60 and 110 mg. per 100 milliliters (ml)) the size of a test tube of blood. Our body's primary source of glucose comes from carbohydrate metabolism, or in other words eating foods rich in carbohydrates, like breads/grains, vegetables and fruits, and beans, which all break down into sugar. Our bodies can in certain circumstances convert other food sources like fats and proteins into glucose/sugar, but the easiest and most direct way to fuel our brains and bodies is by the metabolism of "carbs". Normally, there should be no glucose in one's urine and only a very small amount in the blood stream- that 60 to 110 mg. blood level. This is where the problem lies in DM. Because of the lack of insulin, or either the person's insensitivity to insulin, our body allows sugar to "pass through" to where it should not be, and these elevated levels of glucose/sugar cause damage in our blood vessels, specifically our arteries, by way of the development atherosclerosis. Atherosclerosis is basically scarring & inflammation of the inside linings of our blood vessels, which sets up conditions like clot formation and narrowing of the vessels. This is how you get a heart attack or a stroke. This narrowing of the blood vessels contributes to the development of hypertension, or high blood pressure as well. Sixty (60%) of diabetics have hypertension, as defined as a BP of >130/90. The word sclerosis actually means scaring. It is this narrowing of blood vessels and clot formation is what makes diabetes the trigger to developing stroke, heart attack, peripheral artery disease in the feet and legs, kidney disease, and blindness due to damage to the tiny blood vessels supplying the retina in our eyes. Subsequently, damage to other organs via damaged blood vessels supplying decreased amounts of nutrients and oxygen to them will fail as well.

The incidence of diabetes mellitus (DM) in the US is increasing by truck loads as we speak. Its incidence is not just rising, it is soaring. According to the American Diabetic Association, there are 25.8 million Americans that have DM. This 25.8 million represent 8.3% of the adult US population (ADA, 2011). This number represents an increase of 22% over just 5 to 6 years ago. Of that 25.8 million, 7 million of these diabetic people have not been diagnosed yet. The symptoms of DM do not appear until blood glucose levels run consistently over 200mg/dl. DM is the sixth leading cause of death in the US, but that number is probably higher because that statistic is taken from death certificates and diabetes is not usually listed as the cause of death; but heart attack and stroke more commonly are. It is estimated that diabetes contributes to approximately 250,000 deaths a year. It is a major player in the development of several other diseases. According to the CDC, diabetes mellitus is clearly a factor in the development of heart disease, stroke and high blood pressure. Truly it has made its home in the cardiovascular system, our hearts and its vascular pipeline. It affects all body systems, causing significant damage to our blood vessels and organs. The most life threatening consequences of DM are heart disease and stroke and these patients have twice the incidence of dying of them than people who do not have DM. http://www.diabetes.org/diabetes-statistics/heart-disease.jsp. The chemical reactions of DM cause our blood vessels to narrow, or close up completely. This vessel disease's official name is called atherosclerosis and DM speeds up its progression. Frequently the patients whom I've seen in the OR having heart bypass surgery or open heart surgery due to atherosclerosis (coronary artery disease) or CAD also had DM. The CDC says that DM is associated with having heart surgery 30 % of the time.

Another frightening reality is that diabetes is the leading cause of non- traumatic amputation. Having a limb/leg, a toe, or a foot amputated due to the ravages of uncontrolled diabetes mellitus, with years of elevated levels of circulating sugar is alarming. All of our organs, both big like our hearts and small like the nephron units in our kidneys are oxygen and nutrient dependent upon our vascular systems, that pipe line of tiny arteries that do the job of delivering the life saving blood for their and our survival (i.e., eyes, brain, heart, kidney, little toes, feet, legs and fingers). Consequently, blindness is another major morbidity associated with DM. DM is the acronym for diabetes mellitus used by the medical profession when writing. The blindness caused by DM is a result of impaired blood flow in the tiny arterioles that supply one's retina, the organ of sight that sits in the back of the eyeball. Blindness is a tragic consequence of any disease. The worst part about the blindness caused by DM is that it is not reversible. Once the retina dies, that's it. It is literally "Lights out". The incidence of blindness associated with DM is staggering. According to the CDC, Diabetes is he leading cause of new cases of blindness in adults between the ages of 20 and 74. Likewise, the National Eye Institute estimates that 40% to 45% of all Americans affected by diabetes will develop diabetic retinopathy (fancy word for blindness caused by DM) and that 24,000 of these patients will go blind each year. This statistical prediction is horrible.

Another complication or nightmare of diabetes mellitus as mentioned previously is amputation. Too frequently in the operating room there will be one room that is doing some kind of amputation. At least 50 times in the 10 years I worked in the OR, I've assisted in surgery where a gangrenous limb succumbs to the saw. Yes, they use real Black & Decker saws and other power tools too. Likewise, I know that toes are a common body part affected by DM.

I have a friend who is a podiatrist, a foot doctor and he states he sees at least 50 patients a week for diabetic foot care. Diabetics need to pay extra special attention to their feet because of the poor circulation to the tiny blood vessels in their feet and toes. This is commonly known as peripheral vascular disease or PVD. A diabetic person mandates intensive disease prevention management and care of their feet to prevent the worst case scenario of infection and amputation. I worked for a home care nursing agency for a few years while attending graduate school and I performed diabetic wound care to feet that were ulcerated, infected and almost black with gangrene on a daily basis. What made it easy for me to give this intensive care to their feet was that I never hurt any of these diabetic wound care patients because they could not feel what I was doing, because their feet were numb due to diabetic neuropathy. Diabetic neuropathy means that the nerves died because of the DM. Diabetics are given specific instruction on how to prevent any kind of trauma to their feet to thereby prevent infection. It is important for a diabetic to immediately report any cuts or sores on their feet that become increasingly red, develop swelling, or if they detect any drainage, especially if it looks like pus and or if it has a foul odor to it. Smelly, thick, yellow greenish drainage *always* indicates infection. So if it smells funky call your doctor immediately. If a diabetic patient gets even a small cut or blister on his or her foot, that small cut can, if not kept clean, snowball into a horrific infection, which could lead to amputation of a toe or a limb. Likewise, many diabetics have decreased sensation in their feet due to damaged nerves caused by the diabetes. Therefore, all diabetics need to **visually inspect** his/her feet daily for any sores, ulcers, blisters, or cuts because they might not know that anything is wrong because many diabetics can't feel their feet, because they have no or decreased sensation in their lower extremities. Diabetics need to be instructed to look at their feet daily and check for the S & S (signs & symptoms) of infection. Every diabetic should be under the care of a podiatrist, or foot doctor, and should be seen on a regular schedule to monitor and maintain good foot health. Some examples of the ravages of diabetes that I have witnessed in the OR are as follows: These are worst case scenarios that I would not have believed if I didn't see it for myself in the OR.

I know of a 50 year old morbidly obese overweight 300 pound man to whom this exact set of circumstances had happened. I'll call him John, again. John's history reads as follows. John had no history or was not aware of the disease DM. John accidentally burned the bottom of his right big toe when he stepped onto the hot surface of his fireplace's hearth. His toe developed a blister from the burn. The blister broke and subsequently the open wound became infected. Weeks later while doing the laundry, John's wife noticed that one of his socks was soiled with this foul smelling yellow and slightly bloody drainage.

When she mentioned this to her husband he agreed that he thought his feet were sweating more than usual and that was probably the reason for his wet socks. But John never really looked at the bottom of his infected draining foot and toe. He felt there was no need to inspect it, or look at it. After all, he felt no pain. Days to weeks had passed and he eventually noticed that he had an open sore on his big toe. He decided to treat his toe himself using over the counter medicines, triple antibiotic creams, dressings and wraps, but the toe continued to drain and smell. John's wife was a nurse but John never showed her his foot. John thought he could take care of it himself. A couple of weeks later, John started to feel ill. He began running fevers of 102 to 103. He had these intermittent fevers which he treated himself with Motrin or Tylenol for over a week. He finally showed his wife his foot and she became alarmed at what she saw. She saw a huge open ulcer on the bottom of his toe. The ulcer was full of pus. That night John's fever kept spiking higher, despite his taking Motrin every four hours. It was the weekend and his regular doctor did not have office hours, so he decided to go to the emergency room for treatment. John was immediately admitted to the hospital. His diagnosis was cellulites of his foot/toe and diabetes mellitus. His had a random blood sugar draw of 360!!! (we all know now that normal blood glucose should be under 110). He also was diagnosed with hypertension or high blood pressure, and a severe staph infection of his right great toe. John's BP was dangerously high with a reading of 220/ 120. Self -reporting diabetics report a 67% incidence of high blood pressure (ADA, 2011). His white blood cell count (WBC), which when elevated is an indicator of infection was a sky high 27,000. Normal WBC is below 10,000. The infection in his toe was so bad, it had invaded the bones of his toe and foot, a condition called osteomyelitis. John had no choice but to be admitted to the hospital. The emergency room doctors started him on intravenous antibiotics and the next morning John underwent emergency surgery for the amputation of his right great toe. The doctor said that if they did not remove the infected toe when they did, that John would have developed a more severe blood infection, worse than what he already had, and that it could have been life threatening. John never knew he had diabetes. He also never knew his foot was burned because he never felt any pain, because his foot lost its sensation from the neuropathy from the diabetes. John fell into that pool of 7 million people or 20% to 25% of diabetics who don't know they have DM. It's a vicious circle.

Diabetes is easily diagnosed. There is no fancy or elaborate testing schedule needed to diagnosis DM. There must however be 2 definitive readings of a blood sugar (BS) over 126mg./dl. A person must be fasting for at least 8 hours before taking the blood glucose test. Fasting to the medical community means no caloric intake for 8 hours before. The reason for this is so that the reading will be a true reading without the interference of pancreatic hormones affecting glucose levels. In a normal non-diabetic person with a glucose level under 110mg/dl, his glucose level will naturally spike between 30mg./dl and 40 mg./dl within 15 minutes after eating. This is normal, but the elevation will only be temporary. If this non diabetic person eats before taking the test, his glucose level will reflect a false positive reading 30mg to 40mg over the true value, and his glucose level might register way over 100 mg/dl depending on what he ate. We all know now the normal fasting blood glucose is within 60 mg/dl and 100 mg/dl. Depending upon the fasting 100mg./dl level line to cross, that will determine if a person has DM or not. Now, there are levels of positivism for DM. A fasting blood glucose registering between 100 mg and 126 mg will signify a status of pre-diabetes and of having impaired glucose tolerance. Blood glucose levels over 100mg./dl are not normal (Burke, Sandra, 2009). According to the American Diabetic Association (2006) a fasting blood glucose at or above 126mg./dl is diagnostic for diabetes. This criterion is the rule.

John's story had a happy ending. John recovered after his toe amputation and he is fine today. He keeps tabs on his blood sugar, takes his medicines, modified his diet, and goes to the foot doctor every few months for maintenance diabetic foot care. Also, loosing excess body weight is of crucial importance in managing DM, as obesity is highly associated with the development of DM. This case was a close call. In retrospect, John had many of the risk factors of developing DM. Despite no family history of DM, John did have high blood pressure and he was severely overweight, tipping the scales to over 300 lbs. Keeping a normal weight for your height is of paramount importance in the prevention of DM, as we will see later in this chapter. Fat consumption does not cause you to become fat, high sugar consumption makes you fat.

Not every patient with diabetes will develop complications as severe as this patient. John's DM was what could be considered uncontrolled diabetes. Amputation is a major consequence of unmanaged uncontrolled diabetes. Below the knee amputations frequented our OR schedule way too often. Approximately 1.2 million people in the United States are living with some form of amputation. Of this number, the Agrability Quarterly (2005) reports there are currently 380,000 people whose amputation is of a lower extremity; above or below the knee, ankle, or toes. Below the knee amputations, or BKAs are the most common type of lower extremity amputation. Amputations are due to various diseases and events. Diseases of the blood vessels, commonly known as peripheral vascular disease (PVD) and **diabetes (DM) account for 82 %** of all the amputations in the US. Other causes of limbs being amputated are; trauma 22%, congenital defects 4%, and 4% are due cancerous tumors. So you can see how DM keeps operating room personnel employed. (http://www.healthsystem.virginia.edu/uvahealth/adult_pmr/amput.cfmtocanceroustumors.http://www.healthsystem.virginia.edu/uvahealth/adult_pmr/amput.cfm). Other conditions that may lead to amputations are blood clots, and osteomylitis (infection in bone). John had this bone infection. As noted above, diabetes (DM) is responsible for the majority of leg and foot amputations. My patient John lost his right great toe to DM. Every patient is different with different sets of circumstances. I only document this particular case as I would never have believed it if I hadn't witnessed it with my own eyes. John's story is classic for consequences of uncontrolled DM.

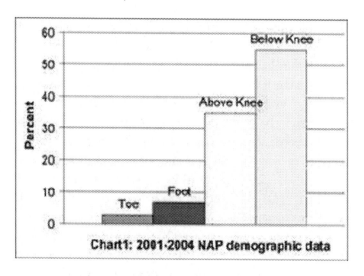

Chart1: 2001-2004 NAP demographic data

Oh No, there is another diabetic amputation story. Ready?

This topic of diabetic amputation brings me to the focus of my next encounter that "I wouldn't believe it if I didn't see it for myself in the OR" case. It was truly a saddest case scenario. To me, it was probably the most physically demeaning, emotionally draining, and psychologically crippling, frightening event to ever happen to a diabetic patient or a person I've ever scrubbed for in my professional OR career.

I was working the 10 am to 6 pm lunch break shift on this particular day. It was 3:00pm and I was scrubbing at the sink to relieve the OR tech who was scrubbed in OR suite #2, the URO suite. I peeked into the room before I started scrubbing and saw that the abdominal case was just starting because the residents were only starting to drape the surgical field. The circulating nurse was hooking up the bovie cord to the cauterizing machine and rolling it into place, close enough to the surgical field so as not to provide a tripping hazard over its cord. I entered the room with my arms bent at the elbows, my hands extended and pointing toward the ceiling. Water was dripping from my pointed elbow joints. The outgoing scrub nurse handed me a sterile towel to dry my hands and I donned a sterile operative gown. I noticed that there was a pungent order that hit my masked face as I walked closer to the operative field. It was not a pleasant scent. The odor was a mix of strong medicine and putridness. I then stepped up one level onto a standing stool and suddenly my eyesight locked directly onto a ghastly nauseating surgical wound. But this surgical site was unrecognizable to me. "What's this?" I thought to myself. There was a definite mound to this anomaly. "What are we doing here?" I asked the surgical resident standing beside me. "This is Mr. Xs infected penis." "Why is his penis infected?" I asked. I couldn't imagine! The resident continued, "He is a diabetic patient. He's only 54 years old. For years he struggled with the medical regime. We can't be sure if he took his insulin shots as instructed. His blood sugar levels were constantly high, above 200. Now, his diabetes was wreaking havoc on his body."

Mr. X had Type II diabetes, which is what most adult diabetics have, 94% to be exact. He developed DM as an adult. Type II DM means that his body makes some insulin, but not enough, or his body is resistant to insulin's effects. Type I diabetes usually initially affects children and follows into adulthood who do not produce any insulin at all, and are dependent upon life long insulin injections. Some Type I diabetic patients opt to use an insulin pump instead of self injecting. Type I diabetes is a genetic condition, but it is not directly or automatically inherited from a parent. The proof lies in the fact that in the case of identical twins, only one of the twins can develop Type I DM, but the other does not. However, there is a genetic component to Type I DM, and it is believed that there is some genetic predisposition, or trigger to its development. Regardless of the type of diabetes, Type I, Type II, or gestational, the consequences are the same if blood sugars are left unchecked. This Type II diabetes develops over many years and then blossoms, usually in middle age. However, statistics show that presently, even children are increasingly developing Type II diabetes as well. According to the ADA, 1 in 400 children and adolescents in the US has Type II DM. That number equals 0.26 % of this population bracket (ADA, 2011). As the American abdominal girth expands, so does the incidence of DM. Type II DM is acquired after a lifetime of poor diet and it is highly associated with obesity. And likewise, childhood obesity associated with Type II DM is increasing, but this doesn't have to be the reality, because both childhood obesity and childhood acquired Type II DM are both completely preventable! **100% preventable!** It is important to note here that the consequences of DM in children are the same as in adults.

The surgical resident continued, "Mr. X's pancreas was just not manufacturing enough of his own insulin needed to control the sugar overload in his system and his cells have become resistant to insulin." Most of these Type II DM patients do not need to inject themselves daily with insulin, but they do need to manage their diets, restricting bad/white sugars and sometimes take some kind of oral hypoglycemic agent in pill form so that they can maintain their blood sugars under 110 mg. Keeping one's blood sugar under 110 can help prevent furthering diabetes's devastating effects of blindness, heart disease, stroke, high blood pressure, PVD and kidney failure to a minimum. Mr. X's now had progressed to this present condition. This patient had it all; he had high blood pressure, he was nearly blind because of the diabetic retinopathy, and his kidney function was almost non existent as he was on hemodialysis three times a week. "So what is he here for today?" I asked the surgical resident. The surgeon replied, "He developed a sore on his penis about one month ago and now it has become infected. The infection he developed is threatening his life. We're amputating his penis, but only partially." "Oh, that's good", I smirked under my mask as I rolled my eyes in disbelief. The surgeon continued, "The patient's infection or type of bacteria has become very resistant to the antibiotics we're using and now there's only one way left to treat it. The only way to approach this infection is to surgically remove the source. Excise it from his body." Well this was a first for me. I had never heard of amputating a penis before! I thought I had seen everything, but this was almost unbelievable. For a split second I thought I was in a horror movie. The odor of the infection was gross. To me this was a worst case scenario, a truly devastating consequence of any disease. Since his infection was running rampant, the only thing left to do to prevent Mr. X from dying of septicemia was to remove the infection's source, **his penis!** This was truly a most tragic event. I thought to myself, "No one is going to believe me when I tell people that this is a possible consequence of DM."

"Pass the specimen bowl please" the surgeon asked me. I passed the sterile shinny stainless steel round 8 oz.

pan to the surgeon. I watched as he carved out the dead glop of flaccid tissue from the patient's pubic area with a fresh # 7 scalpel blade. The tissue, his penis looked to be about 2 ounces in volume. It was unrecognizable as a penis as any lay person or medical professional could identify. It certainly would have fooled me if the urologist hadn't passed it to me and clearly stated what it was. This patient did not have his entire penis amputated, only the distal third. That's enough, don't you think? I say this sarcastically, shockingly and sadly.

The wound was dressed and Mr. X was taken to the RR. I never saw the man awake. You may be wondering how then does this poor gentleman urinate? The answer is simple. Because of his uncontrolled diabetes, Mr. X had developed "End Stage Renal Disease" or **ESRD**, otherwise known as kidney failure. The tiny nephron units in his kidneys lost their abilities of filtering and urine concentration and he was dependent on hemodialysis for fluid homeostasis. Another most unfortunate squeal of diabetes is kidney failure. **88% of ESRD-kidney failure in the US is due to DM**. This case was one of the most depressing moments in my OR career. They taught me these things in nursing school, but I was shocked by how devastating the consequences of DM were when I finally saw it for myself.

I take every opportunity I get to tell everyone I know and love of the perils of having uncontrolled diabetes because it will shave 10 to 15 years off of your life, but only after it disables you or takes your eye sight away from you. But the good news is that many of the complications of DM are completely preventable, most of the time if one can manage their blood sugars. Unfortunately and sadly,

ESRD as a consequence of DM is not reversible-**outside of a kidney transplant!** We do these in the OR too!

Risk Factors for DM

One of the goals of this book is to bring awareness of the prevalence of DM and to help identify risk factors that predispose to its development. The risk factors of DM are everywhere. It affects all ages of all peoples It is important for everyone to identify the red flags and then to focus their behaviors to correct any unhealthy habits. Certain ethnic and cultural populations are more at risk than others. The risk factors I have encountered in these worst case scenarios that have corresponded with known medical research as documented by the American Diabetic Association are listed as follows:

1. Native Alaskan, Native American Indian, African American & Hispanic American peoples. (Mr. X was African American) (John was Caucasian and morbidly obese).

2. Family history, especially if close relative like mother, father, sibling have it. (Mr. X was + for family hx; John was not)

3. Inactivity (Both Mr. X and John had this risk factor)

4. Older than 45 years old. (Both Mr. X and John had this risk factor)

5. High blood pressure. (Both Mr. X and John had this risk factor)

6. Previous diabetes while pregnant and or baby weighing over 9 pounds.

7. Obesity, especially with excessive belly fat, and or BMI (Body Mass Index) of over 25. See below how to calculate. (Mr. X was not obese, but John was morbidly obese and off the BMI charts below!)

8. Blood lab levels of
   a. triglycerides > 200 or
   b. HDL cholesterol < 35.
   c. Fasting blood sugar of >100 signifies impaired glucose tolerance
   d. Fasting blood glucose equal to or over 126 mg./dl is diagnostic of DM. (Both Mr. X and John had blood sugars over 200mg./dl)

Just as important as knowing the risk factors associated with the development of DM, is having awareness of the signs and symptoms of DM. If you notice any of these report them to your primary health care practitioner promptly.

S & S of Diabetes Mellitus

#1 Increased thirst

#2 increased urination

#3 increased hunger

#4 increased lack of energy

#5 a sore that does not heal and or if it looks infected, especially on the foot #6 blurred vision or loss of vision

All are symptoms that need prompt medical attention and can be associated with diabetes, but are not limited to DM. These symptoms could be associated with other conditions. Never try to diagnosis yourself. Just as important as knowing the risks for developing diabetes, know also that **erectile dysfunction can also be a symptom of diabetes.** I know you've seen the TV commercials.

Obesity

Body Mass Index (BMI) has recently been introduced as a means to determine the degree of body fat as it is related to the risk of developing diabetes. Obesity is a major risk factor in the development of DM. The BMI or Body mass index is a ratio of a person's height to weight. It is an indicator of body fatness. It is used as an assessment tool for determining overweight and obesity. It is easy and inexpensive to do. The magic number is **"25"**. As long as your BMI number is around 25, or a little less than or at 25 you're OK. A BMI of over 25, but under 30 indicates moderate overweight. A BMI of over 30 indicates obesity. Morbidly obese people have BMI s of between 40 and 50. The formula used to determine BMI is as follows:

Weight in pounds/ divided by height in inches, squared, and then multiplied by a factor of 703. Please don't ask me what the 703 factor is or stands for. I am not a mathematician or a statistician. It just works. It looks like this:

<u>(Pounds) = (#)2 X (multiply) 703</u> = BMI
(inches)

For example, if someone is 6 ft. 2 in. tall, and weighs 200 lbs, you just divide the weight 200 lbs. by 74 (inches in height), square it(2), THEN MULTIPLY THAT BY 703 and that result equals 32.5. This person's BMI is over 30, so he is classified as obese and is at risk for developing diabetes.

Another example is a woman who is 5 ft. 2 in. tall and weighs 120 lbs. Lets quickly calculate : 120 lb. / 64in. (2) x 703 = 23. This woman's BMI of 23 indicates that she is normal weight and is not a risk factor for diabetes. A BMI table is listed below for easy reference for those of us who are mathematically challenged. This is cool!

BMI Classification ranges are as follows:

> < 18.5 underweight
> 18.5 – 24.9 normal weight
> 25.0 – 29.9 overweight
> 30.0 -40 – obese
> 40-50 morbidly obese

Actuaries, the people who work for insurance companies, will utilize BMI tables in order to classify people into weight categories and correlate this # to determine risk factor assessment for developing certain diseases for insurance billing. A person who is obese will pay a higher premium for a life insurance policy because he carries a greater risk of dying at a younger age, just as a person who is older will pay higher premiums. Or a person who smokes cigarettes will pay more money for his life insurance policy because he is at higher risk for dying sooner due to high blood pressure, stroke, heart attack, or certain forms of cancer. There is to cheating. The insurance companies and their actuaries have it down to an exact science. Plus, the insurance companies will obtain a urine specimen that will reveal if nicotine or some drugs, legal and not are present.

BMI table

To use the table, find the appropriate height in the left-hand column labeled Height. Move across to a given weight (in pounds). The number at the top of the column is the BMI at that height and weight. Pounds have been rounded off.

Select the **PDF** version for better printing

BMI	19	20	21	22	23	24	25	26	27	28	29	30	31	32	33	34	35
Height (inches)							Body Weight (pounds)										
58	91	96	100	105	110	115	119	124	129	134	138	143	148	153	158	162	167
59	94	99	104	109	114	119	124	128	133	138	143	148	153	158	163	168	173
60	97	102	107	112	118	123	128	133	138	143	148	153	158	163	168	174	179
61	100	106	111	116	122	127	132	137	143	148	153	158	164	169	174	180	185
62	104	109	115	120	126	131	136	142	147	153	158	164	169	175	180	186	191
63	107	113	118	124	130	135	141	146	152	158	163	169	175	180	186	191	197
64	110	116	122	128	134	140	145	151	157	163	169	174	180	186	192	197	204
65	114	120	126	132	138	144	150	156	162	168	174	180	186	192	198	204	210
66	118	124	130	136	142	148	155	161	167	173	179	186	192	198	204	210	216
67	121	127	134	140	146	153	159	166	172	178	185	191	198	204	211	217	223

To use the table, find the appropriate height in the left-hand column labeled Height. Move across to a given weight (in pounds). The number at the top of the column is the BMI at that height and weight. Pounds have been rounded off.

Select the **PDF** version for better printing

BMI	19	20	21	22	23	24	25	26	27	28	29	30	31	32	33	34	35
Height (inches)								Body Weight (pounds)									
68	125	131	138	144	151	158	164	171	177	184	190	197	203	210	216	223	230
69	128	135	142	149	155	162	169	176	182	189	196	203	209	216	223	230	236
70	132	139	146	153	160	167	174	181	188	195	202	209	216	222	229	236	243
71	136	143	150	157	165	172	179	186	193	200	208	215	222	229	236	243	250
72	140	147	154	162	169	177	184	191	199	206	213	221	228	235	242	250	258
73	144	151	159	166	174	182	189	197	204	212	219	227	235	242	250	257	265
74	148	155	163	171	179	186	194	202	210	218	225	233	241	249	256	264	272
75	152	160	168	176	184	192	200	208	216	224	232	240	248	256	264	272	279
76	156	164	172	180	189	197	205	213	221	230	238	246	254	263	271	279	287

http://www.nhlbi.nih.gov/guidelines/obesity/bmi_tbl.htm

Waist circumference is also used as a reference as a DM development risk factor because **abdominal fat indicates visceral obesity**. Visceral obesity is defined as the fat surrounding internal abdominal organs. This type of abdominal fat most commonly is linked to diabetes as well as some cancers and heart disease too. According to the American Journal of Epidemiology, June 15, 2008, Researchers have demonstrated that people with high abdominal fat content, as measured by waist circumference of greater than 35 inches in women and greater than 40 inches in men **are 20 times more likely to die earlier than those people who only have an elevated BMI of over 25, but with normal waist circumferences**. When measuring waist circumference, measure directly around and above the upper hip bone.

Obesity here in the United States is on the rise and has been for the past two decades. The Center for Disease Control and Preventions estimates that over 60 million adult Americans, that's 30 % of adults over the age of 20 are overweight (BMI >30). This increasing rate of fatness is alarming because being overweight or obese carries significant health risks for developing severe health conditions that can shorten your life span, and or impact the quality of your life. Diseases associated with being overweight or being fat are:

1. Sleep apnea
2. Dislipidemia-high cholesterol
3. Hypertension
4. Heart disease
5. Stroke

6. Gallbladder disease

7. Osteoarthritis

8. Diabetes type II

9. Endometrial, Colon, and Breast Cancers

But why are we so overweight? Where does the problem or problems lie? Surprisingly, the answer is simple. The underlying cause of obesity or being overweight is due to an energy imbalance. The CDC defines this overweight energy imbalance as the result of the number of calories consumed is not equal to the number of calories used. There are many causes for this energy imbalance. For instance, genetics plays a role in the metabolic clock that determines the rate of metabolism of an individual. Cultural differences can dictate dietary habits that can contribute to this imbalance as well. Recent research demonstrates that clinical depression is also associated with obesity. But the factor that impacts this balance the most is our behavior of consuming more dietary calories than the energy we expend due to inactivity and a sedentary lifestyle. We just don't move like we did a generation ago. We don't walk to the store, we drive to the store. I remember when I was a teenager I walked over a mile to and from my high school to the bus every day. Today, my daughter's school bus picks her up one block away at the corner and takes her to the school's doorstep.

Other factors that contribute to obesity are a sedentary lifestyle and the leisure activities we choose. Computer activities and engaging in social networks and playing video games dominate many of our extracurricular activities. During the past decade the PC has impacted our waistlines as well as our daily activities. Instead of going outside and playing tennis, we play "Pong" on our Play Station. Instead of meeting friends for a game of touch football, we slip in "Asteroids", find a comfortable chair and "Hyperspace" ourselves into oblivion! And don't forget the chips and soda for energy. Here in the US, childhood obesity is at an all- time high. 17% of children and adolescents (12.5 million) from the ages of 12 to 19 years old are classified as obese, which is defined as having a BMI of between 30 and 40 (CDC & NHANES, 2010). Videogames can consume hours and hours of sitting in front of a television or computer screen. Adults and children alike, also find conversing in chat rooms on their computers a favorite activity. Sitting in front of a computer screen has become a routine activity for many of us, as we routinely shop, take college courses, invest, pay bills, do homework, or just surf the web for fun. Facebook, which is a social networking site, is the new favorite pass time and the only thing it requires for you to do is to sit in front of your computer screen for hours!

Our consumption of sugar based products has contributed significantly to this energy imbalance as well. Donut Shops, Baked cakes and cookie products, and fancy flavored white chocolate mocha coffees are my favorites. I've even witnessed a cook from the Food Network channel prepare a recipe featuring a bread pudding made with Krispy Kreme Droughts. Ummm! I heard on the television station CNN last week that Americans consume an average of 175 pounds of sugar a year. That is a lot of sugar. I visually tried to picture how high a mound of 175 pounds of sugar would look like and just for fun, I came up with this scenario. 175 lbs of sugar equates to 35 five pound bags of sugar. That is approximately 2 times my body mass. I did some calculations regarding the nutritional values of sugar that are documented on the 5 pound bag of sugar, then infused some dietary/ nursing knowledge and came to these conclusions:

1. The bag of sugar's nutritional value chart states that 1 serving of sugar is equivalent to 1 teaspoon = 4 gm of carb and provides **15** calories. A calorie is a unit of heat energy.

2. A 5 pound of sugar contains 567 teaspoons or servings of sugar.

3. 567 (tsps) x 15 (calories per tsp.) = **8,505** calories provided per 5 lb. bag of sugar.

4. 175 lbs. of sugar per year reduces to **35** five lb. bags of sugar per year. (175/5=35).

5. those 35 five pound bags of sugar consumed per year are equivalent to 35/12 (months) = eating 2.66 five pound bags of sugar per month

6. If 8,505 calories are in one 5 lb. bag, then 8,505 x 2.66 (bags per month) = 21,513 sugar calories consumed per month.

7. Remember that 3,600 calories = 1 pound of body fat.

8. 21,513 / 3600 = 5.97 pounds of body fat gained from sugar per month.

9. So if you eliminated the 2.66 five pound bags of sugar a month you'll **lose 5.97 (6) pounds just by cutting out the sugar!** Can it get any easier???!!!

10. Likewise, if 8,505 calories per 5 lb. bag, then

11. 8,505 cals x 35 (5 lb. bags per year) = 297,675 calories consumed from sugar per year.

12. 258,156 sugar calories consumed per year /3600 cal/lb = **71.71 pounds of body fat, weight gain per year from eating sugar.**

Now, let's convert this caloric sugar intake into body fat. Everyone's caloric intake varies according to height and age. But, for exemplary purposes I'll use the average.

The average adult requires 2,200 calories to maintain the average metabolic functions. Any excess calories consumed over this 2,200 per day and not expended by exerting energy will be stored as fat for later use. Fat is stored in the body in various places. It can be stored in a protruding abdomen, globules of cellulite in one's buttocks, flabby flesh waving from your triceps, or lumps bulging from your thighs over your chair seat while sitting. One pound is equal to 3,600 calories. Any excess caloric intake of 3,600 calories will equal one pound of body fat. So if our example person consumes 3,600 calories over his required 2,200 (2,200 + 3,600 = 5,800) calories he will gain one pound. Let's plug in our pound values into our sugar consumption.

Regarding item #6, if you consume 21,513 excess sugar calories per month, this can be converted into body fat by dividing 21,513 calories consumed by 3,600 calories per pound and that equals **a 5.9 pounds of monthly weight gain** if not worked off by exercise. The same can be calculated for the yearly sugar consumption of 297,675 calories in 35 five pound bags of sugar. 258,156 calories consumed, divided by 3,600 (calories needed for 1 pound)

= 71.71pounds of weight gain per year, if not worked off by exercise. This mathematical exercise reveals the insidious effects of sugar, weight gain and obesity. These calculations are for eliminating white sugar only and the sugars found in fun foods and processed foods like soda pop, candy bars, and sugar baked products like cakes and donuts and cookies. Natural sugars like sugars found in whole fruits and vegetables are not included in foods to be eliminated. It all sounds too good to be true, and it sounds too easy to be true. I think that sugar has evolved into an addictive substance just as the smoker craves his next nicotine packed cigarette, and the alcoholic shakes his way to his next beer. I hear my mother say from time to time how she "Needs to eat something sweet" even after a hearty meal. There is no scientific evidence of any molecular or genetic dependency, but perhaps we as Americans have developed a cultural dependency on sugar. Frequently we Americans use Sugar /candies as rewards and as gifts of affection. Baking a cake to give to a new neighbor on the block, and gifts of chocolates on Valentine's Day are traditions we hold dear in America.

Despite the pleasure sugar gives us, in excess its effects can be harmful. Sugar control is central in managing diabetes, but we need to take control of our dietary behaviors before sugar's detrimental effects take control of our lives and health. Many friends ask me what methods they should employ to manage their weight. I know there are dozens of books on fancy diets, and even the TV screams with ads selling movie star diets. But the best advice I can give anyone is to count your calories, limit sugar intake and exercise. **The basic principle to weight loss is that your caloric intake must not exceed the**

energy you burn/use via activity. Another prime example of our sugar dependency is our habitual consumption of carbonated beverages. Soda is loaded with sugar. It is packed with 170 calories per 12 oz can. Eliminate it! Alcohol is sugar laden as well. One can of beer contains 190 calories. They call it a **"Beer Belly"** for a reason! And that six pack you chugged down last Friday night at your best friend's bachelor party totaled 1,140 calories. Limit candy consumption as well. One candy bar contains over 200 calories of concentrated sugar. Eliminate it. When you sit down to eat a meal, eat the fruits and vegetables first. By eating these bulk forming foods first, which are lower in calorie content yet higher in fiber and roughage, you can gain the sensation of fullness sooner and by the time you approach the meat portion of your meal, which is always higher in calories and fat content, so you will not eat as much. This approach of eating less food and exercising to lose weight is significantly less expensive than TV advertised diets as well.

Increasing physical activity can combat obesity as well and promote cardiovascular health. The CDC recommends exercising daily with a 30 minute moderate work out 5 times a week (walking), or a 20 minute more intense work out 3 times a week (swimming, running). The most useful web sight used for this chapter is from the CDC. www.cdc.gov/obesity

Here are some practices you can employ to increase physical activity and burn calories, without feeling that you are working out, but you really are:

1. Take the stairs.

2. Park your car furthest away and walk to the entrance of the mall.

3. Take your dog for a daily 1 mile walk.

4. Run the vacuum and mop the floor.

5. Mow the lawn, gardening

6. Do 100 sit ups a day, if physically and medically possible

Glycemic index is another method popular in dieting today as well, and it works. Calculating a food's glycemic index (GI) and applying it to your diet is another method of monitoring carbohydrate intake and its impact on your blood sugar. Carbohydrates are food items that break down into and provide sugar to our bodies for energy. Examples of carbohydrates are fruits, vegetables, and grains. Anything that grows from the soil and we eat is a carbohydrate. More specific examples include, bananas, cherries, oranges, avocados, broccoli, asparagus, corn, tomatoes, pineapples, beans, oats, other grains, beans and wheat (breads). It has been proven that some carbohydrates will cause a large and rapid spike in our blood sugars which is associated with diabetes and obesity, while others will cause a smaller, slower and steady blood sugar elevation. According to Mendosa.com (2006), foods that should be avoided and that cause the highest glycemic responses are "starchy foods" or the "bad carbs".

Examples of bad carbs that cause a rapid spike in BS are:

#1 most sugary breakfast cereals

#2 bread
#3 processed bakery products
#4 baked potatoes.
#5 Candy

Foods that cause a low glycemic response are the "good" carbs and do not cause a rapid BS spike are the better carbs.

Examples of good carbs are:

#1 pasta
#2 oats/oatmeal
#3 beans
#4 brown rice

Surprisingly, according to the GI method, table sugar does not cause a high glycemic response. It is categorized a mid range glucose elevator. Foods are assigned an "index number" based on a blood sugar obtained 2 to 3 hours after eating a specific amount, usually 2 oz. The higher the index number the more likely that food will elevate your blood sugar higher and more rapidly, and it is more likely that food could contribute to obesity and diabetes. The magic number is to eat foods that supply a number less than '**55**' per 2 oz. serving.

The Nutra System style of diet, which is based on this GI, is in my opinion a healthy diet regime that promotes eating foods in moderation; it limits calorie consumption, while incorporating all food groups that supply nutrition, without depriving the person any one food substance. The Nutra System and GI based diets eliminate those super sugary food products that dissolve immediately into sugar as soon as they enter your mouth and produce rapid BS spikes.

Upon examining these styles of GI based diets, I have believe they are easier to use and easier to stick with, because you are not depriving yourself of any one type of food group. Unlike the Atkins diet which practically eliminates fruits and vegetable initially, in my opinion, is not a healthy way to exist, unless you do it for a very short time. The Atkins diet will work, and initial weight loss is rapid, but it is not sustainable, nor realistic. We human beings need to consume fruits and vegetables because eating fruits and vegetables are essential sources of vitamins and minerals needed for all basic metabolic functions. It would be detrimental to our health if we were to eliminate fruits and vegetables. A good argument in favor of consuming fruits and vegetables is the disease Scurvy. Survey is caused by the lack of vitamin C. Scurvy will kill you and it won't take long. Six months tops. Vitamin C is a water soluble vitamin, which means that it dissolves in water and is eliminated from our bodies readily through our urine, every day, every time. It is not stored in our body fat like vitamins A, D, E, and K are. With fat soluble vitamins, our bodies can tap into its fat reserves whenever it needs them. Vitamin C needs to be replenished in our bodies almost daily. Settlers to the new world back in the 1700s died in scores due to the disease scurvy as they lacked the consumption of fruits, and vegetables, specifically the citrus fruits and vegetables that they were used to eating in Europe and did not grow in the new world, or they did not know about. North America's soil and weather is not conducive to growing citrus/tropical crops in the New England and Middle Atlantic states where many of the first immigrants settled. Lemons, oranges, pineapple, avocado, and limes do not grow in Virginia, Pennsylvania, New Jersey, Delaware, New York, or Mass like they do in Italy, Spain, France and Portugal. For more information regarding glycemic index log onto, http://www.mendosa.com/. Another resource used to reference glycemic indices of popular foods is the *Amer. Jour. of Clinical Nutrition*, 1995, vol 62: 871S-890S. This latter source specifies foods and their glycemic indices for easy reference.

The lesson to be learned here is to arm yourself with valuable information you can use to maintain health and prevent disease.

1. Maintain a normal weigh with a BMI of 25 or below.

2. Maintain a waist circumference appropriate for gender: <35 inches for women and < 40 inches for men.

3. Know the risk factors of diabetes

4. Be aware of the Signs and Symptoms of diabetes

5. Report any S & S of infection to your doctor

6. Exercise regularly, walk, swim, isometrics, play sports, dance, vacuum, Hoola-Hoop, or whatever you can do, just move 30 minutes a day.

7. Eliminate as much white sugar & simple sugars from your diet as possible and eliminate processed foods as well. Processed foods contain high amounts

of sodium (salt) which contributes to high blood pressure. If it comes in a package, it's processed.

8. Strive to keep Blood sugar below within normal range of 60 to 110 mg/dl, especially if you are already diabetic or pre-diabetic.

CHAPTER 5

BREAST CANCER

Working as a registered nurse in the operating room exposes oneself to all sorts of medical as well as surgical issues that one would never see or even hear of in the lay world. Sometimes a patient will require a surgical procedure for a medical condition which is seemingly unrelated to the original diagnosis. It seems confusing at first, but after connecting the dots it makes all the sense in the real world. This next surgical procedure is such an example, with a heart wrenching twist.

I was working in the pre-operative area or holding area on this particular day. It was after lunch and by this time the number of operations to be started was dwindling. Typically the mad rush is in the morning when there are 17 cases that all have a 7:00am start time. During the morning surge, the holding area nurse's responsibilities are too numerous to list, but in the afternoon I could now could talk to the patients one on one and attend to their psychological needs more so now as the cases became staggered. The double doors to the OR suite swung open as Curtis, one of the nursing assistant transports entered the vestibule of the OR, wheeling a stretcher with young woman sitting up with her kneels bent. Curtis placed the head of the stretcher against the OR green colored tiled wall. The patient was smiling. She didn't look sick nor did she seem to be in any distress. She had soft curly strawberry red hair, rosy cheeks, and her tiny nose was sprinkled with freckles. Actually, she was the perfect picture of health. I thought perhaps she was undergoing some sort of plastic surgery, maybe even a breast augmentation. Breast implant surgery was beginning to become very popular then. It was the summer of 19XX. As a matter of fact, after years of observing people up close and literally under their skin, I developed the art of picking out what is fake or surgically implanted, or altered, and what was not. I've seen the before and after hundreds of times and every day, all day long for many years. For example, detecting breast implants is as easy as spotting a bad toupee once you realize the direction gravity pulls objects. I could even tell you what kind of operation you had in the past by just looking at your surgical incision's scar. Case in point: We had a neighbor named Carlos, who was bragging about his gall bladder or "cholecystectomy" operation that he had 3 months ago. He was joking to my husband and me about how many stitches his scar had. Laughingly, he pulled up his shirt to count the number of scars left by the stitches. "Sixty eight!" He stated laughingly in a loud voice. I sat there silently, peering at his abdomen. He had no idea that I was a nurse, let alone an operating room nurse; a person who was familiar with practically any kind of operation any person could ever have. "Clearly that was no gall bladder scar", I thought to myself. His abdominal scar ran the whole length of his abdomen from the bottom tip of his sternum down and around his umbilicus (belly button), and then midline down straight to his symphysis pubis (his pubic bone) immediately above his pubic hair line. I knew from experience that this man either had a staging laparotomy for some type of cancer, whereas the surgeon needed to biopsy numerous lymph nodes throughout his abdomen and pelvis, or he had some kind of emergent surgical procedure. Perhaps he was a trauma victim, a car accident victim where the surgeon needed as much visualization as possible to correct a lacerated blood vessel before he bled to death. I could not be sure but I definitely knew he did not have his gallbladder removed, or he had way more than just his gallbladder removed. I did not let on that I knew he was covering up the real reason for his surgery. So, I let it go. I figured that I eventually would learn the truth. Calling someone's bluff in front of others is not a classy thing to do, especially since he was going out of his way to conceal the truth. There was something he clearly did not want me, or anyone else to know. I certainly did not want to invade his privacy which he was obviously struggling to maintain. Lesson learned here: We all have a sense of pride laced with a thread of vanity that we must respect. Carlos was dying and he knew it. Carlos died 9 months later at the age of 56 of cancer. Carlos told my husband, 8 months later, 2 weeks before he entered a hospice that he had been diagnosed with stage IV colon cancer. Carlos died with dignity. The abdominal scar he displayed was a staging laparotomy scar for the staging of his colon cancer. He was a dear man. PS: Carlos is a fictional name, but the person was real.

The young lady who just arrived was still smiling. "Hi, my name is Kathy. I'm the holding area nurse. What is your name?" I asked. "Donna" she replied (Donna is a fictional name, but the person is real. Donna was the name of my best friend when I was a little girl). I touched her left wrist and asked if I could read her plastic ID bracelet. It read Donna XX, Room # 7009, her patient ID #, and NKDA. NKDA is the acronym for no known drug allergies. But just to be on the safe side I asked her more, "Do you have any drug allergies?" "No" she replied. People forget all the time of some quirky drug they took many years ago that caused hives or extreme itching and they treated themselves with Benadryl or did nothing at all, not knowing that those are symptoms of allergy. So I changed my questioning method just to be sure. I needed to get Donna to think of her response and not just go through the motions and answer Yes or No. So I next asked her "Do any medicines or foods cause you to break out in hives or a rash, or does any medicines or foods cause you to have shortness of breath or wheeze or cough? I thought that this type of question would force Donna to think about her answer, and not just give me an answer that she thinks she wanted me to hear. "No, nothing I can think of" she replied. "How about any environmental or chemical items, like latex?", I asked. This is an important question for anyone undergoing the knife. Allergy to latex has been increasing since its documentation in 1979. Latex allergy has been known to cause anaphylactic shock and death. Up to 10% of the US population is allergic to latex. Latex allergy is most commonly documented in people who have a cumulative exposure or many exposures, and latex lives king in the operating room. So many items used in the OR are made of latex, specifically the sterile gloves worn by the surgeons and the surgical team. Interestingly, 10 % to 17 % of healthcare workers themselves have developed allergic symptoms to latex and 2 % have developed occupational asthma as a result of latex exposure. It is believed that this is a result of the snapping of surgical gloves and the subsequent aerosolization of latex particles. The sterile gloves worn by the surgical team during an operation are made of latex. According to the FDA (2008) recent estimates revealed that approximately 22% of health care workers are sensitized to the traditional latex extracted from the sap of the rubber tree, Hevea braziliensis. How people find out they're allergic to latex is when a person wears a pair of latex gloves that they've purchased for protecting their skin from abrasive chemicals like bleach for cleaning or perhaps someone would wear a pair when tackling a painting job and when they removed the gloves their hands are full of welts, or hives and they are itching like crazy! Years later I read how there is a cross sensitivity of latex allergy to fruits like bananas, avocados, kiwi, chestnuts, and tomatoes, as their molecular proteins resemble the latex protein. This is an excellent screening question for peri-operative patients, to ask if the patient experiences any allergy symptoms like wheezing, cough, shortness of breath, hives or itchy rash after eating foods like bananas, kiwi, tomatoes, or avocados as it might signal OR personnel to a potential disastrous anaphylactic reaction to latex and to take precautions to avoid latex. It is interesting to remember that latex is not a manufactured or a chemically engineered product. Latex is a natural plant product just like those above fruits. Latex is the term used for the milky white, sometimes yellow sap of many plants which coagulates when exposed to air. Latex can be tapped from over 63 plants, all found in the Americas. It is farmed from plants and trees grown in the forests of Brazil and other tropical and subtropical countries. It is interesting to note that these fruits, bananas, avocados, and kiwi are all tropical plants just like the plant that makes latex, as they are chemically related and grown in the same soils.

Latex allergy has been documented primarily in people who have a prolonged cumulative exposure to the substance, most notably in the health care industry where latex gloves are routinely used and in patients who depend on medical devices made of rubber, or latex; like urinary catheters, and latex drains used in operative surgical wounds and incisions. Patients who have undergone surgical procedures early in life are also at risk. Ten percent (10%) to seventeen (17%) of health care workers have developed allergic symptoms to latex. Latex allergy did not become apparent until 1979 and it is increasing and is widespread. But good news regarding latex is in the news today. According to an article in the Nursing Spectrum, June 16, 2008, the FDA cleared the first device made from a new form of natural rubber latex –a glove made from the guayule bush, a latex native to the desert of the Southwestern United States. Data from studies of this new product show that even people who are highly allergic to traditional latex do not react on first exposure to the guayule latex proteins. The FDA concludes that the new latex may prove to be a safer alternative for people with severe latex sensitivity. We shall see.

Kathleen E. Volpe-Schaffer RN

Years later when I was employed at a pediatric triage company I received a phone call from a distressed mother stating that her 6 month old infant had developed a red rash that looked like hives all around the baby's mouth. His lips appeared swollen and his breathing sounded noisy and he was coughing. It was clear to me that the baby was exhibiting allergic symptoms, potentially life threatening symptoms as the baby sounded to me like he was wheezing. And this was over the phone! I asked the mother if the baby was allergic to anything at all; foods, medicines, animals, but the mother said "NO, NO, NO to everything". I told the mother that she needed to take the baby to the ER STAT, but it would be better, quicker if she called "911". She said "OK" she would do so immediately. I waited on the phone until the emergency personnel arrived. In the meantime, I asked the mother what the baby looked like and what the baby was doing and she said "He's doing the same thing, he's sucking on his new Binki". I told the mother to take the pacifier out of the baby's mouth immediately, as pacifier nipples are made of latex and that the baby could be exhibiting an allergy to the latex in the rubber nipple. The baby was taken to the hospital by ambulance and it was later determined that the child had an allergic reaction to the latex pacifier. This story is just an anecdotal incidence and is an example of latex allergy and how wide spread it is.

Donna answered "No". I proceeded next to check her operative permit. The procedure that Donna signed for was a "Bilateral Oophorectomy". This operation is the surgical removal of both ovaries. This fact was troubling to me, first of all because Donna was only 32 years old and secondly because it signified to me something terrible and life threatening. Being a nurse I knew that this procedure was her last chance to slow down the spread of a rampant malignancy being fed by the female hormone estrogen, which is produced by the ovaries. Healthy 32 year old women do not routinely have both of their ovaries removed. I flipped through her chart to the pages that were tabbed "history and physical." I was very curious, but I needed to confirm my worst fear. The first sentence read "32yr. old white female with stage III metastatic breast cancer admitted for bilateral oophorectomy." The history went on to describe how her breast cancer had receptors to the hormone estrogen, but the saddest paragraph I read was how her breast cancer had metastasized to her liver and how the organ was studded with cancerous tumors. I hoped she didn't see the sadness in my eyes as I tried to keep a straight emotionless face. I knew this was her last chance for any hope. I continued flipping through the chart aimlessly, only to occupy my emotions and to focus the direction of my eyes away from Donna's. I didn't want to look into her eyes anymore as I was afraid I would start crying. I knew from my formal education that once cancer spread to the liver it was most likely advanced. Her life expectancy outside of divine intervention could be severely curtailed. I thought to myself, "Could this scenario get any worse?" As I continued to read Donna's gynecological history, another gut churning fact was revealed.

"G2, P2, AB 0" read the next sentence. Of course it could! This statement was the worst news. Now I knew that Donna would be leaving two children motherless. In medical shorthand, the G2 meant that her uterus was "gravid" or pregnant twice, and the P2 signified that she gave live birth to two live children, or "Parturated" two times. The acronym AB and the number 0 revealed that she never had a miscarriage or an abortion. These facts were numbing, but I had to continue.

I composed myself and continued with my discussion. I was curious. "Donna", I asked, "Forgive me, but can I ask a personal question?" "Sure", she said. I cleared the frogs from my throat. I really had more than one but I figured if I phrased my question properly I could obtain more. This was the first time I ever saw a woman so young, only 32 years old who had breast cancer. Usually the breast cancer patients I've encountered in the OR were older, much older, and certainly not pre menopausal. As any person knows, the risk of developing breast cancer increases with age. Years ago I remember asking a famous breast surgeon, Dr. Gordon Schwartz MD of Thomas Jefferson University Hospital, "Is there anyone, any woman who does not get breast cancer?" What better person to ask than a breast doctor/surgeon. Dr. Schwartz devoted his whole life to the study, research and treatment of breast cancer and breast diseases. His answer surprised me. He replied to me, "Yes" he said to me "Women who are multiparous (gave birth to 2 or more children) before the age of 18." Well, that was frightening to me, because I didn't have any children yet and I was already 28 years old when I asked him. That statistic hit too close to home as I was included in that oceanic pool of women. But to me his statement also inadvertently revealed to me the answer to the question as to why today breast cancer is more widespread, at least here in the US. Today, women put off having children till their 30's, 40's and insanely in my opinion, until their 50's, whereas & conversely,

30yrs ago and prior to that, women made careers out of housekeeping and childbearing. Think about it. Women in underdeveloped countries who bear children, many children early in life don't have the high breast cancer rates like we do here in the US, if they have any incidence of BC at all. I recently read an article in "Time" where an epidemiologist, Dr. Zheng from Vanderbilt University in Nashvill, TN. claimed that "reproductive changes are responsible for about 30% to 40% of breast cancer risk (Kingsbury, Kathleen, 2007)." When women bear children and breast feed, it is like giving their bodies a vacation against the hormone estrogen. Breast cancer is more common in higher socio-economic areas and it is thought because of delaying child bearing to later in life and having less children, that incidence exposes a woman's body and breasts to more lifetime estrogen. See www. worldwidebreastcancer.com   for statistical information regarding this issue.

Donna was not menstruating as this fact was clearly documented on the chart; 'LMP 0/0/XX", which was 3 months before this date. LMP is the acronym or abbreviation for "Last Menstrual Period", and this date was only last month. This was clearly alarming to me. I probably over stepped my boundaries but I had to know, so I asked…

"What happened? How did this come about, you're so young! I don't understand? And if you don't feel like talking about it, if you feel it is none of my business I'll understand" I added.

"It's OK Kathy. Everyone asks the same thing. I want people to know." My first thought was to ask her when did she discover she had cancer, but without my prying any further she initiated telling me of her plight. Donna started talking openly and calmly. "I noticed this lump in my right breast, here on the side near my armpit while I was breastfeeding my daughter."

"How old was your daughter when this happened?" I asked. "She was only weeks old" Donna replied. "What did you do? Did you tell your doctor?" I anxiously awaited her answer. "Oh yes! I told him when I went back for my six week post partum visit. He even gave me a through breast examination. He told me it was a benign mass; probably related to me breastfeeding. He told me that sometimes the milk ducts get plugged up. He also told me it was nothing to worry about. It was most likely a clogged milk duct." "Was it painful?" I asked. "No, not at all" was her reply. Before I go on, I have to tell you of a story I read in a magazine article on breast cancer a few years back. A physician had a female patient who came to him presenting with a breast cancer that had erupted through to the skin. The physician asked the woman how long she had this wound, and when, and if she ever felt a lump. The patient replied that "Yes she did feel a lump" and the doctor asked her how long ago she noticed it. She said she noticed the lump approximately 17 years ago. Next he asked her, "How come she didn't come in earlier to report it?" Her answer was, "Because it didn't hurt". Breast cancer does not hurt. So if you feel a painless mass or any lump, contact your primary health care provider promptly. Also, as any woman who has ever breast fed knows, when you get a clogged milk duct it is usually extremely painful.

"How big was the lump? Was it pea sized, grape sized or walnut sized?" I asked Donna.

"It was large grape sized" was her reply.

"Was the lump hard or squishy?" was my next question.

"It was hard" she answered.

Was there any blood in your milk supply?" was my next question. "None" was Donna's response. I thought about asking her if she noticed any discharge at all from her nipples, but I realized that that was a stupid question for me to ask because she was breastfeeding. Of course she was. So I stopped with the blood from the nipple question.

I felt weird asking these personal questions but I felt compelled to do so. In my mind I was going through the laundry list of sings and symptoms of breast cancer that I wanted to ask. "So what happened next?" I asked. Donna said, "Nothing happened. I continued life as usual. But the lump kept getting bigger."

"Did you call to tell your doctor that it was getting bigger?" I asked.

"Oh yes. As a matter of fact, when I went back for my six month check up (4 ½ months later !) I told him again and he still insisted that it was benign and that it was still related to me actively breast feeding." Her response floored me, but I kept a straight face. I then asked, "Did your right breast look any different from the other one, like its size or shape?"

"Not really" she said.

"Did the skin over the lump and or breast look as it normally did, or was it like, smooth or dimpled?"

"It did look like it was pulled", she replied.

"Did anyone else in your family ever have breast cancer?"

"No, no one."

"That's it" I thought to myself. She had definite indications of possible advanced stage breast cancer, for months, maybe years, and she didn't even know it. She was lead to believe that everything was OK when it wasn't. I was getting angrier by the second. I feared that this cancer would kill her. I knew in my heart that barring any miracles, her life would be shortened. **In 80% of BC cases there is no family history**!

"Well, when did someone do something to discover that it was cancer? When did someone do a biopsy or order a mammogram or an ultrasound?" I continued asking questions.

"When I went back for my one year checkup, after the birth of my daughter, I saw another doctor from the same practice and she immediately sent me for a mammogram. The rest is history. I had a breast biopsy and then 10 days later I was scheduled for modified radical mastectomy. They said I had 16 positive lymph nodes in my arm pit. The cancer had spread to a few lymph nodes but the extent to other parts of my body was not known. The chemo shrunk the tumor at first, but not anymore. I'm just doing all I can to help myself live longer. I have two young daughters, you know." I knew.

Donna continued to tell her story. Her two children were 3 and 5 years old now, and Donna was 32years old. That scary statistic Dr. Schwartz told me so long ago came back to flood my conscious. I was having a nightmare and I was fully awake. His words haunted me as I realized Donna was an example of her not being included in his sample population of women who don't get breast cancer. But really, who is? Not many of my acquaintances. Donna had her first child at the age of 27. One of the risk factors for breast cancer is having your first child after age 35, but Donna did not fit that risk pool either. The American cancer society lists risk factors for developing breast cancer, but Donna did not fit into any of their criteria. The age of her first period was 12, never took hormones or BCPs, no family history of breast cancer, and she was not overweight. Recently it has been reported that taking BCPs (birth control pills) reduces the risk of breast cancer development. She denied other risk factors as she did not use alcohol and she even breast fed both of her children for months which decreases the number of menstrual cycles thus limiting the amount of hormone exposure. She did everything one should and could have done, except wait. The only risk factor Donna had was being female. My own risk factors for getting breast cancer were higher than Donna's as I didn't have any children yet and I was already 30. Donna then went on to tell how her husband and daughters went to Disney World this spring. They had a great time. It was the first time her children had visited Disney World and it was Donna's dream to do so before she died; to take her two little girls to Disney World as the family she hoped they would always be. She emphasized the fact that she could not stop living. She wanted to live her life to the fullest, especially for her children. She wanted her children to have great childhood memories of their mommy, and to remember all the fun things they did. She said they took lots of pictures and video; a keepsake I'm sure they will always treasure. I'm glad they documented those memories on camera and video.

Her children will always be able to look back to that time when mommy was with them. I thought to myself that they'll need to cherish those childhood memories and to hold on to their mother's image. Long term memory does not develop until the age of four. Her younger daughter would probably have limited memories of her mother or of the trip at all, because she was only 3 years old.

For one of the rare times in my life, I was left speechless.

Upon closing her chart I noticed the royal blue charge plate that was taped to the cover of her chart. I visually scanned all of her personal identification and information that was embossed onto the plastic. Something familiar caught my eye. I stared at the plate for a moment before realizing that Donna lived in the same town I did. Our hometown is not a very large town. I was sure I had never seen her before. "Kathy, please, come see me when this is over", she pleaded. The doctors had told her she would be home by the weekend so we made a date for the next Saturday. I was attending a university on a part time basis and working full time so that weekend was a perfect time for me to visit. At that moment the anesthesiologist appeared, asked a few questions and proceeded to roll Donna into the operation room.

I kept my date and I went to visit her 5 days later. I met her family, her husband and children and her parents. Her children played and laughed as normally as toddlers would. Donna looked great. I would have never guessed she had abdominal surgery a week before if I didn't see it myself. I was relieved that my visit was purely a social visit, as I found it highly unusual that no one asked me any medical questions. Ordinarily, if people know I am a nurse, they deluge me with a flood of questions. The fact that her family asked me absolutely nothing medically oriented spoke volumes to me on how they were coping with her illness. I instinctively knew that they were fully aware that there were no more questions to ask. There was no more advice to be gotten. Donna was always very cheerful, but with her family and parents I constantly sensed a degree of urgency. There was visible tension on their faces. I would visit frequently over the next three months. Donna never complained about anything. She took care of her children like every mother did, every day. I never heard her state that she was in any kind of pain.

In June of that year, Donna's mom called me to tell me that Donna was admitted to the hospital. That Wednesday after work I went to her room to visit. I entered her private room. Donna said to me with a big smile on her face "Hi Kathy." Her voice sounded weak and raspy. I was horrified when I looked at her. Her body was unrecognizable. Her usual petite 120 lb frame was now bloated to nearly 170lbs. Her abdomen was a mile high as it was filled with ascites, a clear sign that her liver and or kidneys were failing. She looked 20 months pregnant. Her mom and dad were present. I knew that this had to be devastating for her parents as Donna was their only child. Can this story get any more depressing? The anguish was very apparent on her mother's face. Donna had an intravenous in her arm, and she had a urinary catheter to drain her urine. Her hospital room was cool and dark as the vertical blinds were completely drawn shut. We talked about the weather and other nebulous things, stuff that nobody really cared about. Our voices just filled the air. I only stayed for thirty minutes or so. In my last moment there I thought of something happy to talk about. I told Donna I had good news. I told Donna, "The Saturday before I found out from my doctor that I was pregnant." Donna started coughing. I could hear the fluid in her lungs. She then asked me, "What is the baby's due date?" I could tell it was an effort for Donna to speak. I told Donna it was February 14th of next year. I wanted to cut my visit short as I could see it was taxing for her to speak. She was absolutely short of breath. I found that if I held my breath I could hold back the tears. I could tell that she was very happy for me. Donna never stopped smiling. I was off from work the next day so I told her I would visit the day after tomorrow, during my lunch break. I kissed her head said good buy to her parents and left. Two days later when I returned to her hospital room, I walked into a sun filled empty room. The vertical blinds were wide open and the room was in the process of being terminally cleaned by the housekeeping personnel. I immediately ran to the nurse's station and asked the dreaded question. "Where was Donna?" The charge nurse turned to me and stated "She died early this morning. The undertaker took her body about an hour ago." I went back to her sun drenched room, approached the open window and just stared out into the cloudless blue sky. The sunlight was blinding. It was a beautiful day.

This was my first up close encounter with a person I knew personally and her family battling breast cancer. In Donna's memory and in every other woman's memory who battles breast cancer I shall always empower every woman with the knowledge needed to combat this disease.

A few days later while driving passed my church, the same church Donna and her family attended, I noticed that he parking lot was full of shinny black cars with hot pink funeral stickers affixed to them. It was Donna's funeral. For that moment I slowed my car down to a coast, looked over at the flower laden hearse that would carry Donna's remains to their final resting place, swallowed, and then continued on. I was torn because I had tickets to a graduation, but I didn't care about graduation anymore. I knew my family would be totally pissed off at me if I pulled a stunt like not showing up, so I said a Hail Mary, blotted my tears and continued on.

Donna's mother told me months later that Donna's husband sued the gynecologist who delayed addressing her breast mass for almost a year, for $250,000. Donna should have been ordered by that first physician to undergo a mammogram when she first discovered the lump, or at least to get a second opinion from another physician. That's my opinion. If a mammogram had been performed when she first detected the lump and the cancer discovered just a year earlier, her life expectancy could have been quite different. She would have had a chance. Early detection could have saved her life. Instead, she wasted a year of guessing and watching her breast cancer grow. At the very least, her physician should have ordered a mammogram after her second visit to him, as she was still complaining of the same breast lump, which was now increasing in size. Clearly, it was at this point where that physician failed his patient. That initial physician essentially made too light of her symptoms. He attributed the mass to breast feeding and a clogged milk duct. He just assumed that because of her age that it was a benign mass related to her breast feeding. It is true that a woman's chances of developing breast cancer increase with age, but that is no excuse to assume that younger women don't get breast cancer too, because they do. Although 75% of all breast cancers occur in women older than age 50, younger breast cancer victims, those under the age of 40 develop larger and more aggressive tumors, like my friend Donna. Death rates for younger breast cancer patients are higher than for the over 50 age group. According to CDC (2008) breast cancer statistics, whereas 85% of breast cancer patients in the 50 to 69 year old age group will be alive in 5 years after diagnosis, only 80 % of the women ages 30 to 39 years will be alive in 5 years after diagnosis, and a gloomier mere 72% of the women aged 20 to 29 years old will be alive 5 years after diagnosis. Those statistics scream the importance of not taking lightly any breast mass, especially in a younger woman because if the mass is a breast cancer, it is more lethal to her. Being a physician, he should have known. This is my opinion. Let it be known that overwhelmingly most breast lumps in younger women are benign. My intention is not to scare women, just to be informed. Only 7% of breast cancers are diagnosed in women under the age of 40.

The lesson learned here is to get a second opinion if you have any doubts, but more importantly it is imperative for all women to be pro active and to arm yourself with knowledge. So many of us are tainted by breast cancer, whether it be a mother, a sister, an aunt, a grandmother, or a friend. I believe all women, including girls beginning at the senior high school level become informed about the risks, and signs and symptoms of breast cancer. I think that all high school senior girls should be taught the correct method for performing self- breast examination

(SBE), despite recent recommendations that SBEs be done only yearly by a physician. The school nurse would be a great resource for this subject. This knowledge base of SBEs, or at least obtaining risk factor information should be included in the senior high school health curriculum, just like sexually transmitted diseases are taught. The message here is to tell women to "know your breasts". Know what your breasts look like, and know what they feel like, and if you notice a **change**, call your health care practitioner.

What makes death by breast cancer so tragic is that it is an unnecessary death, because there are screening methods available that make its early detection easy, and if caught early, BC treatments claim a success cure 95% of the time. This is a fact that should empower women to just do it- Get that yearly mammogram, have your primary care practitioner do a yearly breast exam, do your monthly self breast exams, be aware of the risk factors, and communicate with your doctor and you'll sleep better and live longer. I drag my 80 year old mother to get her mammo. She's full of excuses from it gives her a headache, to it gives her gas, which I know is bologna. I know she's a fraidy cat, as most of us are, so I remind her that she should be more afraid if she didn't get one. A mammogram can detect a breast lump on average 1 to 3 years before it can be felt. By the time a breast cancer grows to a size of 1 centimeter, the size of a pea, it has been growing for 5 to 7 years and is not palpable. A mammogram would most likely detect this size mass instantly. To all those women who are afraid of a mammogram, I propose here and now, to all women, that you should take a "gal pal" on a date to get your yearly mammogram. It could be your mom, your sister, or your best friend. Just go together and you can support each other and you'll have less anxiety. Also, the internet is a gold mine of information, so just Google in breast cancer. The American cancer society provides a wealth of information from risk factor lists, breast cancer disease process with pictures, signs and symptoms, surgical options, drug therapies, chemotherapy, support groups, and anything else about breast cancer. Another sight I used to put together this chapter is the "Breast Cancer Resource Center". It has tons of information also. It is interesting to know that breast cancer is the leading #1 cause of death in women aged 40 to 50, so don't fool yourself. See below BC incidence as correlated to age:

The most common breast cancer statistic you have probably heard is that "1 in 8 women will develop breast cancer in their lifetime." What it should really read is "If everyone lived beyond the age of 70, 1 in 8 of those women would get or have had breast cancer." This statistic is based on everyone in the population living beyond the age of 70. Since your breast cancer risk increases as you age, your lifetime risk changes depending on your age:

Age 20-29: 1 in 2,000
Age 30-39: 1 in 229
Age 40-49: 1 in 68
Age 50-59: 1 in 37
Age 60-69: 1 in 26
Ever: 1 in 8

Source: American Cancer Society Breast Cancer Facts & Figures, 2005-2006.

Chapter 6

Fear

More Breast Cancer

It was 1973 or 74, and I was in my first year of nursing school. I was barely 18 years old. I and my fellow nursing student classmates had been book schooling for the first 6 months and we were now very anxious to begin the clinical "hands-on" part of nursing. We had been practicing making beds (I don't think they do this anymore), how to give injections using oranges, and applying dressings to fake surgical wounds in anticipation for our first real life patients. I was to arrive at my assigned unit, "5 North" as it was called, in the old wing of the Medical College of Pennsylvania, on Henry Ave., in Philly at 7:00 am. It was rumored that the 5 North nursing wing was haunted, and when I arrived and saw it with my own eyes, it looked like it truly was, and for years. It was dimly lit and very chilly. It even smelled cold and musty. The walls were lumpy plaster that nicked and flaked off easily if you banged into them hard enough. The 5 North unit was located in the old original stone building that was built in 1889. As I passed the entrance to the unit, I noticed several patients sitting in big yellow fake leather plastic chairs lined up outside of their rooms. I smiled passively as I walked past each one of them. No body responded to me. My mentor, a real registered nurse whose name escapes me, so I'll just call her Mary, was sitting at the nurse's desk sipping her morning tea. She greeted me, offered me a cup of tea which I declined, and then she proceeded to give me report on the patient assigned to me. "Kathy" she said, "Your patient today is going to be Ms. X. Come with me and we'll talk as we go." Ms. X is a fake name. I do not remember my first patient's name, but her image is plastered in my memory. I got up and walked along side her as we proceeded to the patient's room. Ten seconds later we entered Ms. X's room. "She's a DNR", my mentor said. "What's that mean?" I asked. Mary began her report to me. I learned immediately that **DNR** is the acronym for **DO NOT RECUSSITATE**. Ms. X laid there crumpled in her bed with her head hanging down and bent to the right from a semi fowler's position, and drooling. Her eyes were open, but they were not looking anywhere. Her arms and legs were sprayed in all directions. A foley catheter bag barely filled with intensely concentrated dark yellow urine laid on the dusty dirty floor. I realized immediately that my very first patient was a terminal cancer patient, and was going to die, despite any care, especially from me.

As Mary slowly and gently began to pull the bed sheets down from around from Ms. X's neck, she continued,

"She's a breast cancer patient that was never treated. She walked in too late. The state of Ms. X's breast cancer is the result of total neglect, or just plain ignorance until it was too late." Now remember, this was 1973. Ms. X felt a mass in her left breast and either dismissed it or was too afraid to do anything about it. At that time, mammography was in its infancy, as the equipment specific to performing mammograms did not appear until 1969. Official recommendations regarding mammograms did not exist yet. She never told her husband, her doctor, any friends, or anyone until the cancer ate through her skin and chest wall. She hid her draining breast wound for months. She was only 42 years old. Whether she was embarrassed, or just afraid we'll never know. Mary continued, "When she finally went to the doctor he documented that she had an open fulminating stage IV breast cancer. There wasn't even enough breast tissue remaining on her chest wall left to do a mastectomy. When she came to us, all we could do was to debride the wound and treat her palliatively; keep her hydrated and comfortable. The cancer has already metastasized to her liver and brain and bone. She was immediately terminal. She never had any radiation or chemotherapy, nor any therapy at all for her breast cancer." I just gulped.

Mary pulled down Ms. X's top sheet and removed Ms. X's gown in order to start her dressing change. She had a huge puffy kling dressing over her left chest area. "We're going to change her dressing now. Go wash your hands. We'll do it together now, then tomorrow you'll do it." Mary laid out a chux cloth and then opened the sterile peel pack dressing and flipped them onto the chux. My hands were donned with disposable latex gloves and ready to do my first authentic dressing change. Mary gingerly pulled the paper tape which fastened the dressing to her chest, until the fluff dropped away from Ms. X's chest wound. Immediately, the stench of infection filled my head. I could almost taste it. Diarrhea smelled more fragrant than this virulent infection. The wound was awful and the sight of her malignant chest cavity was even more gross. The baseball sized wound looked like a plate of scrambled flesh. There was no skin to cover what was left of her pectoral muscle. The gaping depression seemed to flow with rivers of color. Purulent streams of violet, mustard black and of course blood red, along with small pieces of adipose tissue stained the old dressing. We irrigated and redressed her wound in less than 10 minutes. But to me, it seemed like hours. I was horrified. Ms. X just laid there looking aimlessly at the ceiling, staring into space as we changed her dressing. Her only response was a slight whimpering when the tape was pulled away from her emaciated bony torso. She never spoke.

This was my first experience with a cancer patient, let alone a dying cancer patient. This was a worst case scenario. I thought to myself, "Could it be any more profound, or any more extreme!!!???" I think not. This patient is an example of what doing nothing can do. At the tender age of 17 -18, an adolescent myself, seeing this monster case of breast cancer instilled such fear in me that I thought every woman who got breast cancer died of it, and in a similar manner. I don't even think that I ever heard of breast cancer before. I can only imagine how in years past this scene was not so rare, and is probably why today women feared it so much. To many women, having a mastectomy is viewed as mutilating, and rightly so. In my opinion I believe they feel it robs them of their womanliness and their sexuality. It alters their identity. Some women can feel incomplete because they feel an integral piece of their female equipment is missing. When I first started working in the OR, in 1978, I only always saw the "radical mastectomy" as the surgical treatment for breast cancer. Today, these radical procedures have scaled back and if a breast cancer is found early, women have choices as to the kind of surgery, lumpectomy vs. mastectomy, combined with radiation and /or chemotherapy, and/or hormonal replacement therapy without compromising her odds for survival. Finally, you can keep your breast if the cancer is found early enough. When the surgeons started doing lumpectomies vs. the mastectomies I was so relieved. My fear factor dropped from a 1,000 to a 5 on a scale of 1 to 10. I saw first hand that the lumpectomy is much less mutilating than the mastectomy. It was quicker and the patients would have much less discomfort after the surgery. I realized that you could even wear a bathing suit with confidence and security.

Case in point: My friend Brenda went for her very first mammogram 10 years ago at the age of 55. She had already been menopausal for 8 years. Brenda said she felt confident that her mammogram would show no cancer, because she would do monthly self-breast-exams (SBE) and she never felt anything abnormal. Her breasts always felt the same; soft, not painful, no lumps in her breasts or armpits, or thickening of any tissues; nor did she ever notice any nipple drainage. Brenda had no family history of breast cancer in her family either, so she felt confident that everything would be fine. A common myth that needs to be dispelled here is that you won't get breast cancer if there is no history of it in your family. In fact, 80 % of breast cancers occur in women with no family history. That's most breast cancers. Brenda fell into this oceanic statistic. Only 20 % of breast cancers carry a genetic component.

Two days after her mammogram she received a phone call from her gynecologist, the doctor who wrote the prescription for the test. He told her that the mammogram showed something suspicious in her right breast and she needed further tests. Another enhancing mammogram showed the possibility of a cancer, so a biopsy was scheduled to test the area in question for cancerous cells. The biopsy was positive for cancer. The size of the lump measured a tiny mere 5 millimeters, barely the size of a match head. A lump this size is not palpable, meaning it cannot be felt by physical examination. Most palpable breast cancers are discovered by the woman herself when she discovers a breast lump. Her surgeon told Brenda that since her tumor was so small and in its early stage, she would be a good candidate for the breast sparing lumpectomy procedure, followed by radiation therapy, rather than the mastectomy which removes the entire breast, but leaves the underlying chest muscle intact. The lumpectomy would only remove the tumor, as well as some surrounding tissue and spare the healthy breast tissue beyond the tumor's borders. Research has demonstrated that these two procedures, lumpectomy vs. mastectomy are equal in outcomes under similar circumstances. Mastectomy is usually reserved for breast tumors that are larger or if there are several tumors in the breast. It didn't take long for Brenda to decide on lumpectomy with several weeks of radiation. During the breast biopsy procedure Brenda had a sentinel lymph node tested for cancer cells, and happily it was negative for any cancer cells. Sentinal node biopsy is a common procedure that is done that only requires one to three of these sentinel lymph nodes to be biopsied instead of the 30 to 40 regular lymph nodes removed in an axillary node dissection. The sentinel nodes are the lymph nodes in the breast that drain and are the first nodes to receive fluids and cells-cancer or not from breast tissue. If one of the sentinel nodes is biopsied and no cancer cells are detected, then the surgeon will probably only do the less invasive sentinel node biopsy and a lumpectomy. This procedure negates the need to have many lymph nodes removed and biopsied, thereby eliminating any swelling or edema of the arm on the affected side. The type of breast surgery, mastectomy vs. lumpectomy will always be determined by your physician. We were all relieved that Brenda's cancer had not spread beyond the breast. Brenda underwent a CT scan of her entire body, and that also confirmed there was no metastasis to any other organs.

Like I said, that was 10 years ago. If Brenda had not had that routine mammogram that detected her breast cancer at an early stage, her experience with breast cancer could have been very different. Today Brenda lives happily with her husband and family in southern New Jersey. The operative words here are **"She lives."**

Desperate Measures

Nothing scares a woman about breast cancer than seeing someone you love afflicted with it. While I was working the holding area in the operating room I encountered an unusual alternative to breast cancer treatment; a prophylactic mastectomy. A young woman aged 35 arrived late in the afternoon at the end of the OR schedule. I checked her chart and read the words "prophylactic bilateral mastectomy with reconstruction" on the consent form. I was afraid to ask this patient any questions because the consent form told me all I needed to know. But it wasn't what it seemed. This patient did not have breast cancer. But her sister did. Her sister died at the age of 38 due to breast cancer. She told me she saw her sister die unnecessarily and she was determined that this was never going to happen to her. This patient was so afraid of ever getting breast cancer that she decided that her only solution would be to have her breasts removed. She reasoned that if she did not have breasts, she could not get breast cancer. That was the first time I had ever heard of prophylactic mastectomy being an alternative treatment for possible breast cancer (?). So I researched it; I just had to know!

To my surprise it was true. Having a bilateral prophylactic mastectomy is an accepted therapy for those women at increased risk for developing breast cancer. That 20 % of breast cancer patients are the women who carry the genetic component-a breast cancer gene- that increases their risk of developing breast cancer to much more than the remaining 80% who do not have the gene. These potential breast cancer patients are truly candidates for this procedure. What causes these 20 % of women to have this higher risk are those who carry the BRCA1 and BRCA2 gene mutations. It is inherited and it is responsible for the family history side of breast cancer. Generally speaking, a woman who lives to 90 years old has a 12% life time risk of developing breast cancer. But a 90 year old woman who carries the BRCA1 or BRCA2 gene mutation has a 60 % to 85% risk of developing breast cancer in her lifetime. This difference and increased risk is huge. In a study done by Klijn, et. Al. (2004), they concluded that breast cancer risk was reduced by 93% by having a prophylactic double mastectomy. But if you opt not to have your breasts removed there are non surgical options. Women with confirmed BRCA1 and BRCA2 gene mutations can be monitored closely by yearly MRI scanning, digital mammography or ultrasound to detect early breast cancers. Tamoxifin and or other medicines can also be prescribed as they can reduce breast cancer risk by 50% in high risk women. Consult your primary care physician and breast cancer/surgeon specialists to see if you are a candidate for this procedure.

Breast Cancer Risk Factors

Having a BC risk factor does not necessarily doom anyone to develop breast cancer. **A risk factor is just a probability score that identifies commonalities** in breast cancer patients. There are many women who have several risk factors and never develop breast cancer, and conversely, there are many women who do not have any risk factors, yet they develop breast cancer. I believe that being informed is better than not being informed and knowledge can empower you to save your life.

1. Age. 75% of breast cancers are diagnosed over the age of 50.
2. Menarche (your period) before age 12.

3. Age at first live birth >30

4. Breast cancer among 1st degree relatives, i.e. mother, daughter, sister

5. Previous breast biopsies. This risk is not associated with the procedure, rather the reason for the biopsy.

6. Race. White women are at greater risk than black women, but black women have a greater risk of dying of the disease.

7. Alcohol consumption !!!! ???? What's this? Read on.

Environmental Factors Contributing to Breast Cancer

#1. Alcohol consumption

One action women can do to reduce their risk of developing breast cancer that I found in my research is to limit alcohol consumption. Dr. Richard Doll, an epidemiologist revealed in the 1950's that women who consumed 2 to 3 alcoholic drinks a day had an increased risk of between 20% and 30% of developing breast cancer (BC). Yes, it has been known for half a century that there was a link between the two; Alcohol consumption and breast cancer. When I did the research on lung cancer for this book and read several of Dr. Doll's research papers-from the 1950's, I was shocked to read about the breast cancer/alcohol consumption link! In the last ten years I have witnessed research confirming Dr. Doll's findings.

As recently as last year the American Cancer society suggested that 11% of the 2009 breast cancer diagnoses were alcohol related (British Medical Journal, 1954). Another scary finding is that researches have determined that there is no minimum level of alcohol ingested that could be considered safe or without risk, according to Naomi Allen PhD, Oxford University, 2009. Even a daily glass of wine bumps the risk up. Even more interesting is the fact that the kind of alcohol consumed makes no difference either, so there is no type or brand of alcohol consumed that is better or worse. All alcohol appears to contribute to BC's development. If you don't believe me,Google it.

Men can get breast cancer too. I encountered 2 men in my OR career who had mastectomies and lumpectomy due to breast cancer. So guys, if you notice a lump in your breast, or unusual nipple discharge, thickening or swelling of a breast, or pain, or any unusual change in your breast, contact your doctor for evaluation. The treatments for male breast cancer are the same as for women.

#2 Obesity

Obesity as related to breast cancer risk is complicated. In a study done at Cornell University in 2008 it was concluded obesity affects BC risk differently at different times of a woman's life cycle. It was noted that obesity, as defined as BMI >25 before menopause actually decreased BC risk development but conversely BC risk development increased with BMI >25 after menopause. Body Mass Index (BMI) is a better indicator for obesity than weight alone. Maintaining a normal weight and BMI are paramount to good health in general, and life time obesity especially well into adulthood in women has been known to be associated with higher BC risk as estrogen is stored in fat tissues and it has been known for decades that having a longer exposure to estrogen automatically increased BC risk. In conclusion, obesity has been documented to increase BC risk in post menopausal women and likewise obesity has been associated with many other health risks. Therefore, maintaining a BMI of 25 is the optimal.

#8 Abortion ? : read chapter 10!

CHAPTER 7

AIDS: I SAW IT FIRST!

Orientation of a new nurse to the operating room takes time. You cannot expect a nurse to function independently for at least 6 months. It was 1978, and I had already been functioning independently for probably almost a year. Operating room nursing is not taught in nursing schools, and if there was any exposure of the nursing student to the OR, it was only for a day or so and then again the student's participation was restricted only to observation from a distance. Sterility of the surgical field is imperative and without extensive technical professional training there would be too much risk to the patient. There is no room for any mistakes. So in the beginning of my OR nursing career, after I attained the basic skills and techniques mandated for independence, I was frequently assigned to minor surgical cases where my nursing supervisors knew I could do no harm. Small general surgical procedures are the norm for the initial experience of specialty rotations before I would progress to more highly technical, lengthy and complicated surgical procedures, like open heart surgery or major orthopedic surgeries. Frequently I found myself assigned to these "General Surgery" small procedure rooms. Inguinal hernia repairs, biopsies of skin lesions and breast masses, hemorrhoid removal, and an occasional appendectomy filled my work day for months. I knew that my skills had to be perfected before I could advance to more difficult cases.

It was during 1978-79 when I noticed an increase in a particularly weird surgical procedure being performed on young men. I would enter the OR's nursing manager's office each morning to obtain my daily assignment only to discover that I was working, again, with a full day of "Fulguration of Anal Condylomas." My OR suite or room would have between 5 and 8 of these procedures assigned to it during an eight hour day. Fulguration of anal condyloma translates into layman's terms as "burning off warts from one's anus." This is just what I wanted to look at all day long (not!). This seemed unusual to me as this kind of surgery's incidence had jumped from hardly ever to regularly needing a full OR room suite at least once a week. "What the hell is going on" I would think to myself. Perhaps I was naive, I was only 23 or 24 years old at the time, but it took some joking from a male OR tech that made me realize what was happening. On this particular morning, Skip, an OR surgical tech, laughingly said to me in his insensitive arrogant macho demeanor, "Hey Kath, are you in that "Fag" room again?" 'Oh my God' I thought to myself, 'He was right!' I knew what he meant. "Oh, shut up Skip" I pretended he didn't bother me, but he did. I knew from nursing school that condyloma, AKA warts, on anyone's genitalia were referred to as "Venereal Warts" in the medical profession back in the day when

I went to school. Venereal warts or anal warts fall into what is known today as a "sexually transmitted disease" or STD. The term "Sexually Transmitted Disease" was not invented in the early 70's when I went to nursing school. We just called it "VD" or whatever it was. Syphilis, Gonorrhea, Chlamydia (the clap), or trich; it was all VD. I think using the term of having "VD" gave an extra nasty kick to the name. It was funny to say. I think to myself today, "Yea right, at least back then VD didn't kill you. All you needed was a little penicillin." Oh wait, yes VD can kill you. Syphilis can kill you. Before penicillin many people died of it. I remember when I was working at MCP in the SICU I had a patient who had to have his mitral valve (heart valve) replaced because his syphilis infection made its home in his heart and the infection scared his mitral valve. If it were not for the invention of artificial heart valves this man would have died of heart failure. Whether the patient was male or female their (warts) location determined if they were sexually transmitted or not. The realization struck me like a bolt of lightning, that these young men with anal warts were in fact homosexual and were experiencing a sexually transmitted disease. VD! Anal condyloma or warts, are viruses that are transmitted sexually. All warts are viral infections, and are extremely contagious. They are passed on by skin to skin contact. Warts on one's genitals are especially contagious and are transmitted readily during sex. But you probably already know that. Common sense also told me that if these patients were contracting venereal warts through anal sex, they had to be getting other forms of VD as well. Gonorrhea and syphilis came to the forefront of my mind. Being a registered nurse and having an education which focused on anatomy and physiology, I instinctively knew from my studies that the human anus/rectum is not genetically engineered for sexual intercourse, despite its convenience. It is not anatomically similar to a vagina, although some people think it is. Not all holes are created equal. A vagina was designed for intercourse and childbirth, and will stretch somewhat easily to accommodate a 7 to 10 pound baby. The rectum will not, or should not, without consequences. The rectum's function is defecation, or the expulsion or stool. Poke a hole through or rip someone' s rectum and they can be dead of septicemia in 72 hours due to the seepage of fecal contents or E-Coli bacteria into one's sterile abdominal cavity. Additionally, the vagina does not (or should not) ordinarily bleed with intercourse; conversely the anus almost always will. It is true that blood born diseases can be transmitted via vaginal intercourse, like hepatitis B & C, HIV, and syphilis, but they are not transmitted as frequently and as readily as rectal intercourse because of the direct transmission of an infectious agent automatically injected into the blood stream through tears in the anal/rectal mucosa. The trauma of rectal intercourse will most certainly open an entry portal for any blood born disease, of which there are too many to list, and with each and every thrust and tearing of rectal/anal tissue. These facts are good causes for using condoms for both women and men regardless of sexual orientation, and regardless of the os chosen.

The surgical procedure of fulgurating the anal warts was to me "unbelievable"...I would not have believed it if I didn't see it for myself, and over and over again. The procedure is done using local anesthesia, so the patient is fully awake. The patient is first positioned belly side down on the OR table and then the table is "jack-knifed". That means that the buttocks are at the apex as the table's and the patient's legs are dropped and then spread slightly apart. The patient's head and chest are only dropped slightly and is kept pretty perpendicular. The patient is given a pillow for his head as his comfort was also important. Next comes the prep. Benzoin, a sticky adhesive liquid is painted about 2 inches long and 2 inches from the anal opening on each side of the anal buttock opening. Then the nurse (me) assists the surgeon in securely placing a 3 inch wide cloth tape to the sticky benzoin solution on each side of the anus and then pulling the buttocks apart while extremely opening the anal os. Each piece of tape is then securely fastened to the bottom underneath of the metal OR table. The anal os is opened to the size of a small lemon, about 2 inches in diameter. The visualization of the anal canal with its flowering warts was now achieved. I use the word flowering because of the way these warts appeared. They made a formation that looked like rose petals encircling the os or opening. They did not look like the warts we get on our fingers or hands or feet. These warts did not look like any wart I've ever seen. These warts stood up on their edges, like circular discs standing on edge in a dish rack.

The surgeon did the usual prep of the area with the betadine solution. I next assisted the surgeon in administering the local anesthesia by holding the bottle of lidocaine with epinephrine upside down and steadily in my hand while the surgeon plunged the sterile needle into its diaphragm and withdrew the needed amount. The next part of this procedure would never cease to give me the hee-bee-gee-bees. The surgeon would then inject, very slowly, into the rectal tissue the numbing lidocaine solution into various sections the patient's anus, at the root of the warts with that 2inch long needle. Sometimes I could feel my own ass pucker as I watched. After a minute or two, to assure that the patient's operative field was void of sensation the surgeon would start the fulguration. With the bovie or cautery knife in the surgeon's hand he would strategically carve out the warts like a woodworker whittles driftwood. Ten minutes later the patient's anus was free of the condyloma, or papilloma or wart, at least on the surface. But we all know now that warts are viruses and viruses are very difficult to kill. Viruses must live on a host or another living creature. They do not live in the air or on inanimate objects, at least for very long. The virus that caused these genital warts is the Human Papilloma Virus. The human pappiloma virus or HPV for short is the virus that causes cervical cancer as well. The HPV numbers 60 strains. There are 20 types of HPV that infect the genital tracts of both men and women. HPV #16 and HPV #18 are linked to invasive cancers of the cervix, vagina, anus and penis as well. http://www.aidsinfonyc.org/hivplus/issue3/prevent/std.html. Oh yes, I said the penis as well. I saw a young man aged 30 have his penis amputated due to a cancer of his penis that was probably caused by the HPV. I had never heard of this ever happening and if it didn't happen on my watch I would have never believed it. In about 50% of all penile cancers, HPV is found associated with it. He was not my patient, but I was consulted regarding his care at that time. I was shocked to learn of this condition. Cancer of the penis is pretty rare. The American Cancer Society predicted approximately 1,200 men got penile cancer in 2009. That statistic translates into about 1 penile cancer per every 100,000 men. There are several risk factors contributing to penile cancer. The primary risk factor associated with penile cancer is **not being circumcised, soon after birth**. It is thought that by not being circumcised, these men develop a condition called phimosis and it is the tightening of the foreskin, and that makes it difficult to retract and keep the area clean. If the foreskin is difficult to retract, a build- up of secretions called "smegma" can develop and this substance can be irritating and cause inflammation. This inflammation sets the ground work for cancer's development. Also, a man's age is another risk factor. 80% of penile cancer patients are older than 55. Having AIDS is another risk factor as well as smoking cigarettes. This medical condition is another reason to use protection when having sex to prevent disease and infections.

Interestingly, Syphilis is often associated with human papilloma virus, the virus that causes venereal warts. Syphilis is a bacterial infection which is also is a blood born disease. Co infection between anal condyloma (warts) and syphilis is common, as with all other STDs. Condyloma that are associated with syphilis have a characteristic shape. They are flat, broad disc shaped, and not rounded like most people are used to seeing. The warts these men had absolutely resembled this syphilitic description. I learned shortly afterwards from a surgical resident, that frequently the patients who had anal condyloma, also had co- infection STDs, like syphilis.

All of the warts that were burned or excised from each individual patient were placed in a 4 oz. sterile plastic specimen jar and sent to the pathology lab. The pathologist's examination of the warts would be the true story. It is worthy noting here that all specimens obtained from any and every patient, regardless of how benign the doctor thinks the tissue specimen appears to be, is always automatically taken to the pathology department for full tissue analysis. No one ever guesses.

In later years, I often wondered how many of those young men were HIV positive and went on to develop AIDS soon after. After all it was 1978 when I assisted with these procedures. AIDS also is a blood born disease, a viral infection and is transmitted in exactly the same way in which these young homosexual men contracted their anal condyloma (anal warts) and perhaps syphilis. In retrospect, they were all probably HIV positive, but no one knew it yet. We know now that the incubation period of AIDS, the period between contracting the infection to when any symptoms develop is approximately 10 years. The acronyms HIV and AIDS were not invented yet. If AIDS was around, and I believe it probably was present, perhaps scattered cases popping up randomly in the 1970's, but not enough numbers to see a pattern forming, it was not detected. It would be another few years before enough numbers, weird untimely deaths, rare & unusual diseases and infections erupted that we would realize that there was a bigger problem sitting immediately under our noses. A new pandemic was in the making. It was just simmering. There was never any "Gay Plague" as some people would incorrectly call it; It was The Plague, only different.

Not long after the anal condyloma rush, about a year later, another weird phenomena occurred in our operating room. There was a plethora of young men in the Philadelphia community who developed a strange and deadly pneumonia. These apparently young healthy men were practically dropping dead from this disease's course. The usual antibiotics used for treating their pneumonias were not working. The doctors needed an accurate microbial diagnosis so that an effective and specific antibiotic or therapy could be prescribed. Sputum cultures and bronchoscopy washings were performed and used to collect specimens to correctly diagnose the culprit. It was mystifying. But they needed more, so there was only one way left to obtain enough lung specimen to sample. So the doctors determined these patients had to undergo open lung biopsies, so adequate amounts of lung tissue could be plated for microscopic examination to try to identify more specifically the microbe responsible. The samples would be tested for sensitivities, or to test what medicine combinations and drugs would be effective in killing it. An open lung biopsy is major surgery. These young men underwent major thoracic (chest) surgery to have samples of their lung tissue excised. Surprisingly, it was revealed that this new and unusual strain of pneumonia was not caused by the usual bacteria, viruses or microbes we were used to seeing. At that time, the most common infectious organisms cultured that caused pneumonia here in the United States were the pneumococcus bacteria, the streptococcus bacteria, hemophilus influenza, and sometimes the tuberculosis bacilli commonly known as TB. Alarmingly, it was discovered that the culprit of this new deadly pneumonia was a relatively benign microbe called pneumocystis carrini, otherwise known as PCP. But why was this otherwise harmless microbe causing such a resistant and deadly pneumonia???? Before 1980 the PCP microbe was not known to cause such a virulent lung infection, let alone death. The PCP microbe is widespread in the environment and normally lives in the human body without any consequence. It was known that sometimes cancer patients who are on chemotherapy or bone marrow transplant patients, both of whom have suppressed immune systems were the only people who were at risk for developing this rare PCP pneumonia. But these young men were otherwise healthy. The medical community was asking, "Why?" For some unusual reason the PCP microbe was multiplying unchecked and became a killer for these young men. This PCP pneumonia was touting a 70% morbidity. Upon further investigation as to why these people did not recover like most other healthy young adults, and the reason as to why they could not fight the pneumonia, it was discovered that this group of patients lacked enough of the specific white blood cells, the T4s, to effectively kill the bacteria, or at least keep it in check like people with normal immune systems could. The usual penicillins prescribed for the most common types of pneumonia were not working. Nothing was working. The victims of this deadly pneumonia just got worse and then died. Initially, when AIDS appeared on the scene, PCP pneumonia was responsible for 50% of AIDS's deaths by causing respitory failure. Then another puzzle piece to this disease was discovered; overwhelmingly, these people who were dying of this mysterious disease were male homosexuals. I guess that's where the tag "THE GAY PLAGUE" came from.

It was 1980-81 and everyone in the OR knew that there was this deadly condition that no one knew anything about. The nurses and the OR techs as well, were all hesitant to participate with these "Open Lung Biopsy" patients. It was very anxiety producing. It seemed to be secretive as well when one of these cases was to be preformed. The procedure was never put on the OR schedule; rather it just appeared, usually crashing through the OR doors. These patients would instantly be transported into one of the OR suites, accompanied by an anesthesiologist and other people whom I have no idea who they were, and bypassing the usual holding area admitting process. What was frightening to us was that no one was 100% sure how this disease was transmitted. There were no volunteers to assist in these operations. My fantasy world worked overtime. I wondered if I touched a patient's hand will I later succumb to this mysterious disease. But I thought "Probably not; not too many deadly diseases are transmitted through the skin." I couldn't think of any. But maybe if it's transmitted via the respiratory route, like the smallpox virus or the chickenpox virus, yes, then I'm dead because there's no vaccine for it. What if the patient coughed on me? That would be the more likely mode of transmission since pneumonia is a respitory ailment. Or maybe it is blood borne. What if I dropped or fumbled with a scalpel that was used to excise the biopsy specimen and I cut myself. Getting sliced by a scalpel would definitely transmit any microbe directly into my blood stream, because the cut would certainly be deep as I would juggle to try to catch it. A scalpel blade is so intensely sharp that at least it would be painless. Most times when you are accidentally cut by a scalpel you don't realize it until you see your glove filling up with blood. These scenarios rolled through my thought process and it scared me. I just prayed that I would not be assigned to one of these "Open lung biopsies." No one ever did ask me. As it turned out, a few brave veteran souls volunteered to staff these rooms where the open lung biopsies were performed. It is important to note here that no one that I know of ever caught anything from these patients in our operating room. But it is equally important to state that we as hospital personnel were just as anxious as the public at large concerning this deadly unknown disease, and especially since we didn't know 100% how it was transmitted. So how could we prevent it? The hospital's answer was to mandate that Universal infectious precautions be used when operating on these patients and all patients until we knew what we were dealing with. We just had to assume that every person who entered the OR was a dirty case. We had to assume that all were infected.

Soon afterwards, in 1981, the CDC published the emergence of an immune deficiency disorder affecting primarily homosexual males and then intravenous drug users. Thankfully, through its diligent research, this scientific community rapidly made ground breaking revelations regarding this plight. We learned how this virus, called the "Human Immunodeficiency Virus" or HIV for short, attacked the immune system, therefore rendering our bodies' immune systems unable to kill the microbes that were causing these unusual and weird diseases, like the PCP pneumonia. Everyone now knows that this PCP pneumonia is otherwise known as an "Opportunistic Infection". Opportunistic infections are the hallmark symptoms of AIDS. An opportunistic infection is caused by an otherwise harmless microbe, but one that takes the **"opportunity"** to multiply and cause disease because the immune system is broken and cannot fix it. The HIV causes AIDS by destroying the T4 cells in our immune systems so that we cannot fight those otherwise harmless infections like a healthy immune system is supposed to do. Yeast infections or uncontrolled thrush is another opportunistic infection afflicting AIDS patients. The T4 white blood cells in our immune systems are responsible for combating yeast /fungal microbes. The connection was made. The microbe PCP has a controversial taxonomy as recent molecular analysis of its mitochondrial DNA revealed that it has an affinity **for fungal stain and therefore the PCP organism is currently classified as a fungus.** It was thought as recently as 5 to 10 years ago to be a bacteria. The mode of transmission of the PCP fungal lung infection is via inhalation of cysts, via the respitory system. But the important fact to remember is that if you do not have HIV, or are not immuno-suppressed, you won't develop PCP pneumonia. The most important aspect of this disease that we learned in the OR was discovering its mode of transmission. Bitter sweetly, I breathed a sigh of relief. Now we knew how to protect ourselves, because the HIV was transmitted via the blood!!!! AHHHHHH!!!!

Other opportunistic infections besides PCP that can be associated with HIV infection/AIDS are: Tuberculosis (TB), Toxoplasmosis, Salmonella infection in the bloodstream, Candida (thrush) and cytomegalovirus just to name a few.

This new disease named AIDS or "Auto-Immune Deficiency Syndrome" was a blood born disease, meaning it is transmitted via the blood route. Likewise, the scientific community discovered that the culprit was a virus. They named this virus the human immunosufficiency virus, or HIV for short. You couldn't get it by kissing or touching someone's skin. Nor could you contract it by the air borne or respitory route. That meant you **could not catch** it by coughing or sneezing in someone's face. This was good news. But being a blood borne disease is not good news for a person working in the operating room, like surgeons, OR scrub nurses, circulating nurses and OR techs, and the housekeeping personnel who had to terminally clean the OR rooms (which involved wiping up blood) after each operative procedure. OR personnel lived in blood, other people's blood, all day long blood, every day blood, blood, blood, blood. We were exposed to blood in more ways than one could imagine. Blood could and would spray out of surgical wounds at any time. I've read where hospital personnel contracted AIDS by blood splattering into the eye. Everyone now had to wear goggles over their eyes and or face shields as protection in case of blood splatter. A single droplet of blood placed on someone's conjunctiva could transmit the HIV infection. Our eyeballs are very vascular and they are capable of absorbing and are permeable to viruses and other microbial infections. Not only can the AIDS virus be transmitted via blood splatter into the conjunctiva, the infected blood splatter could transmit the HIV virus if it made contact with a fresh open wound, like if you cut yourself shaving that morning.

Since the CDC affirmed that AIDS was a blood borne disease and could only be transmitted by blood to blood contact, or if the virus was injected into your bloodstream like via a blood transfusion, it made so much sense that the high incidence of AIDS in homosexual men who practice anal sex, and intravenous drug users, specifically those who shared needles, were dying of this syndrome.

However, early on and interestingly there was also a sobering statistic that most heterosexual or straight people chose to ignore, or probably deny. It was known that in 1981 there was a small less than 1% incidence of AIDS in both heterosexual men and women who were not intravenous drug users. This small statistic clearly revealed the fact that not only gay people got AIDS, but that anyone could get AIDS. Anyone with two synapsing brain neurons could deduce **that this was not a "gay plague",** but rather "THE PLAGUE". This virus could have the potential for wiping out entire populations. This early foolish assumption and denial by the populations at large that only "GAY" men got AIDS probably cost hundreds of thousands of lives. In 1981, I remember attending a mandatory inservice regarding this new disease. The speaker stating explicitly that on that day, there were "450 ? " known cases of AIDS in the US. She really didn't use the term AIDS, but she said some other term referring to the lymph system. She then proceeded to break down the statistics. She stated how this new disease, or syndrome, overwhelmingly affected homosexual males. But this speaker somberly continued that "There was a number of IV drug users who were not homosexual and who were affected with the virus as well.". "Humm", I thought to myself, "This sounds fishy." She kept emphasizing that the homosexual community was primarily at risk for developing this horrible deadly condition, and how homosexual men topped the list of those who were the people being affected. Then she proceeded to state a rather sobering fact. She revealed that not all of the AIDS patients reported in her numbers were homosexual men or intravenous drug users either. She stated **that hemophiliac patients were in that pool of people who contracted AIDS** too. Hemophiliacs receive blood transfusions frequently to control their hemophilia. I thought to myself again, "But not all hemophiliacs can be homosexual! So, no way can AIDS be a gay disease!!!" Then she went to explain that there was a "handful of heterosexual non IV drug users, and a few heterosexual women as well who got AIDS." The number 3 stands out in my mind. Mistakenly, people still focused on AIDS as being a "GAY" disease, when in fact it was not. But no one knew about Africa yet. Today we know conclusively that HIV infection is a viral infection caused by the Human Immunodeficiency Virus which gradually destroys the immune system resulting in infections that are very difficult for the body to fight. Today we know that HIV infection is a chronic medical condition that can be treated, but not cured. There are effective therapies for preventing complications and delaying, but not preventing progression to AIDS.

An accidental AIDS/HIV case comes to mind that demonstrates how HIV when given the opportunity will infect anyone regardless of anything. I say accidental because this person died of AIDS because of blood tainted with HIV before there was testing for the HIV organism. An accomplished tennis star named Arthur Ashe was experiencing chest pains and underwent open heart surgery in 1983. He received a unit of blood as a consequence of the surgery. Mr. Ashe was not homosexual, nor did he do drugs, intravenous or otherwise. Nor was he a hemophilic, but like an unsuspecting hemophilic patient needing a blood transfusion from that era, he died of an AIDS related pneumonia exactly 10 years later, after his HIV infected blood transfusion. That's one statistic I found to be alarming during this book's research. As of 2001, over 14,000 people contracted HIV/AIDS infection via infected donor blood transfusion. Many of these people received blood transfusions that were not tested for HIV, as the testing was not invented until 1985. The first screening test for HIV infection was licensed in 1985. But currently, because of the HIV screening of blood donors, the incidence of HIV transmitted via blood transfusion has been greatly reduced.

Back to Africa; A short time later, it was about 1983-85 the world's worst fears materialized. Several countries on the continent of Africa, where it is believed AIDS originated reported the emergence of a "wasting disease" that local peoples called "the slim". The "slim" resembled AIDS and eventually it was confirmed that it was. The African countries of Zaire and other sub-Saharan countries claimed they had communities with **AIDS populations that exceeded 25 %.** "WHOA!" That figure clearly represents more than any AIDS numbers any where else in the world! That number represents an entity at epidemic proportions. But the most alarming fact that was revealed was that the primary mode of transmission was heterosexual male to female, and vice versa hetereosexual intercourse and not homosexuality. I knew in my heart that his fact proved finally that AIDS was not a gay disease. The nightmare had arrived. Just when was anyone going to fess up and admit that there was a problem, and that 25 % of their country's population was suffering from a deadly unknown disease? Why was this health problem kept secret from the rest of the world and for so long? By 1985 everyone knew that AIDS was truly a pandemic or worldwide event. Just when you think things can't get any worse, they did. The CDC at this time also revealed that the incubation period of AIDS can be as long as ten years. A decade is a long, long time of not knowing that you are carrying a lethal disease and not feel sick at all, and worst of all spreading it to hundreds and perhaps thousands of unknowing souls. One can just imagine the exponential compounding effect that just one single sexually active person carrying the HIV can have in that span of time. The numbers can be phenomenal. I cannot imagine a number that large. No wonder everyone during the late 1980s thought they had AIDS. The sexual revolution of the 1960's and 1970's was over. As of today in 2011, over 34,000,000- thirty four million people worldwide are living with HIV/AIDS, and over 30,000,000 million people have died of AIDS since record keeping in 1981 (UNAIDS, WHO, UNICEF, November, 2011). Today, in 2011, there is an estimated 33.4 million people worldwide living with HIV/AIDS, but 20 % don't know it yet. It's far from over.

This was all wonderful news for employees working in the OR. (NOT)! In our line of work there was always some kind of contact with blood. It came with the territory. It went from being an occupational hazard/nuisance to a life terminating and career altering choice. We had all been exposed to blood for years. Our operating room immediately instituted universal precautions. Now we had to assume that every patient entering the operating room had not only AIDS but every other blood borne deadly pathogen as well. My goodness, I had sneakers stained with splattered dried blood from hundreds of OR patients. My Reebok sneakers probably could test positive for HIV and hepatitis B, C, and D, over and over again as well. Eventually, in 1985 there was the development of a blood test that was able to detect the presence of the HIV that was causing this HIV. Everyone was afraid of having a HIV test. You finally had a reason to be afraid of your past. If you took a HIV test you lost 10 lbs. over the next week waiting for the test results. It took that long. At that time and presently it still is optional for patients undergoing the knife to be tested for the HIV virus. I read an article in the Philadelphia Inquirer on September 22, 2006, that stated the CDC is recommending HIV, AIDS testing for all Americans between the ages of 13 and 64. The CDC recommends that hospitals, clinics, and doctor's offices offer testing so as to detect and initiate treatment modalities in order to delay the development from HIV to AIDS and thereby curb the AIDS epidemic. The CDC estimates that there are 1 million people In the US who are HIV positive, but 250,000 have not been diagnosed yet. Early detection is imperative so that positive outcomes of prompt treatment are attained. If an individual is diagnosed late in the course of the disease, even with standard AIDS treatments that person can extend his life expectancy by 14 years. People with recent HIV infections have a better outlook. These recently diagnosed people, when given standard AIDS treatments can extend their life expectancies by 25 years.

The AIDS patient I remember most vividly was a 20 year old young man I met during the summer of 1983. He arrived to the holding area of the operating room looking as if he had just seen a ghost. His face was unusually colorless. He clutched his blanket tightly around his neck so that I only saw his face. I asked him the usual pre -op questions, but when it came time for me to check his ID band he hesitated to show me his wrist identification bracelet. He slowly and almost painfully exposed his left wrist out from under the blanket, revealing only his left hand and just up to the clear plastic wrist bracelet. This behavior seemed odd. It was apparent to me that he was hiding something. I read his operative permit and then it became clear to me why he was acting as he did. The consent was signed for a skin biopsy, but of what region on his body of skin it did not state. I asked the young man "what was being biopsied?" He lifted the blanket that was covering his torso and replied "THESE." My eyes nearly popped out of my head. His naked chest and abdomen revealed approximately 50 dime to silver dollar sized dark red and purplish irregularly shaped lesions swarming his bony body. Some lesions were raised and blotchy and others were flat. His shoulders, arms, hands, and as far down his thighs as I could see had these lesions also. "OH", I said, "What does the doctor think these lesions are?" "It's Kaposi's sarcoma, a skin cancer", was his reply. I remember how I had read that Kaposi's sarcoma was an AIDS related disease but I had never seen it before. It was my first encounter with this condition. My next question was the most stupid question I ever asked a patient. I questioned him out loud, "I wonder why it only affects your body but not your face. Your face is ivory white and without a trace of any kind of blemish. I wonder why?" I was really thinking out loud. What a mistake that was! "Oh no, it's worse on my face. I look like a monster", he replied as tears started teeming down his face. I was baffled. I gave him a few tissues to dry his tears and he next told me how he has a friend who is an actor, and he gave him stage make up or "pancake" as it is referred to in the acting profession. "Pancake make up covers everything", he told me. "My face used to be beautiful but now I am ugly. I have AIDS. I'm going to die. I know it", and he started crying again. He looked at me with his beautiful large glassy brown eyes and he told me in a soft, almost whispering voice "I'm afraid." Huge tear drops were dripping from his chin. The glacial tears made streaks down his face and I started to see a purplish blotchy hue. The monster part of his disease was peeking through. I instinctively put my arms around him and held his hand tightly. At that point I realized that I had embarrassed him. I was unknowingly insensitive to his plight. I failed nursing 101. As tears welled up in my eyes also, I told him I would pray for him. At that moment the anesthesiologist arrived and whisked him into the operating room. I never saw him again, nor do I remember his name. He would become another AIDS morbidity and mortality statistic. He was probably one of the first patients included in those early calculations that determined the path of this AIDS syndrome. There were no AIDS cocktails or medicines yet. Back in 1983, if you were diagnosed positive for the virus, you knew it was only a matter of time until your life was cut short. All treatments were palliative in the early eighties. Today in 2012, an individual can test positive for HIV and remain relatively healthy, living full lives for decades if not scores. At this writing there is a plethora of drugs that can keep the virus dormant and as many people can attest to, a person can live a near normal live span. Today according to the Henry J. Kaiser Family foundation 11/09 the BBC reports that there is a decline in the number of new HIV infections and it is attributed to education and disease prevention programs according to the AIDS epidemic update 20092009 AIDS epidemic update. As of this writing in 4/2010 the incidence of newly infected HIV has decreased by 17% over the past 8 years.

Kaposi's sarcoma (KS) emerged early on in the AIDS scene. Kaposi's Sarcoma was one of the first AIDS related cancers reported in Zaire in the 1970's, but it was too early to connect all the dots. It was a rare disease before AIDS and was only seen mainly in older men of Mediterranean decent, Jewish and Italian. http://www.nlm.nih.gov/medlineplus/ency/article/000661.htmhttp.

Typically, it is rarely lethal and is routinely a very slow growing cancer, taking 10 or 15 years to develop. KS is really a cancer of the connective tissue affecting ligaments, tendons, bone, fat, muscle, blood vessels, and cartilage. KS usually only appears as one small lesion on the lower leg, sole of the foot, or hand, but because of the immunosuppression of the AIDS virus, AIDS patients develop many lesions and they can be alarmingly disfiguring. KS rarely metastasizes to other organ, but in the AIDS population it rapidly grows and spreads to the lymph glands, lungs, and GI tract. When KS spreads to the gut it become lethal, where it does its most damage by causing bleeding which is the fatal pill. AIDS related KS would routinely have extensive lung involvement that would prove to be lethal as well when AIDS first appeared 30 years ago. But with today's modern treatments of

AIDS related infections, these medicines usually prevent advanced KS from developing. People who have undergone transplant surgery have an increased risk of developing KS as well due to the immunosuppressive therapy needed to prevent organ rejection. But transplant related KS only affects the skin and is easily managed and rarely fatal.

The lesson learned here is to arm yourself with information and take preventative measures to avoid HIV and STDs in the first place. We know so much more today than we did 30 years ago. We know now today that the HIV virus is found in the body fluids of infected persons. In order to become infected with HIV your body needs to have the virus deposited in sufficient quantities by means of semen, vaginal secretions/fluids, blood, or breast milk into your bloodstream. Sweat, saliva, urine and tears do not contain sufficient amounts of the virus to become infectious, or to cause HIV infection. **HIV is not transmitted by routine household exposure** like toilet seats or by kissing. According to the Center for the Study of Aids (2010) the most common mode of transmission of HIV is by unprotected penetrative sexual contact with an infected partner. Contact with infected blood is also a mode of transmission, i.e. blood transfusion. However, since 1992, all blood products administered by health care institutions are screened and tested for HIV. The direct blood route mode of transmission is the most common mode of transmission here in the US is by intravenous drug users who share infected contaminated needles. HIV can also be transmitted from an infected mother to her unborn child during pregnancy and at birth, and through breast feeding. This maternal to child transmission is also known as (MTCT). But progress has been made in reducing MTCT transmission to infants due to the initiating of retro viral therapy to infected mothers.

On the continent of Africa, where the emergence of HIV is believed to have originated, HIV/AIDS is transmitted primarily via heterosexual intercourse. AIDS in Africa is more prevalent in the sub Saharan or southern regions of the continent and is more heavily affected by AIDS than any other region in the world. The world is not out of the woods yet. Despite the decline in new infections According to the Associated Press/Wall Street Journal sub-Saharan Africa is responsible for 71% of new HIV infections recorded in 2008 (Associated Press/*Wall Street Journal* reports (Cheng, 11/24). It is estimated that 24.5 million people were living with HIV at the end of 2005, and 34 million this past year in 2011. In just the past year AIDS in Africa has claimed an estimated 2 million people and more than 12 million children have been orphaned by AIDS, according to UNAIDS 2006 report on the Global Aids Epidemic. AIDS and HIV infection prevalence differs vastly between regions. For example, in Somalia and Senegal the HIV infection prevalence is less than 1%, whereas in South Africa and Zambia 15% to 20% of the adult population is infected with HIV.

Since there is no effective vaccine against HIV available yet, instituting preventive measures remains the best and only means of not contracting HIV/AIDS. Avoiding risky behaviors like sharing needles and having unprotected sex are key factors in preventing HIV infection. According to the Center for the Study of AIDS, practicing safe sex means making sure not to get anyone else's blood, semen, vaginal fluids, or breast milk in one's body, and vice versa for one's partner. Other and more simpler ways of prevention are to:

A. practice abstinence
B. limit sex to a faithful monogamous relationship with an uninfected partner.

Advice here is :

1. Think before you act.

2. Use condoms. Think of your partner's health as well.

3. Have yourself tested for HIV. If you test positive, know that modern therapies with the HIV retroviral treatment medications can stop people from becoming sick for many years. These antiretroviral treatments work by combating the HIV infection by slowing down the viral replication process in the body.

Antiretroviral therapy for HIV very often is a combination of 3 or more medicines. These medications are recommended for HIV positive patients who are faithful and committed to taking all of their medications and who have a CD4 blood count of between 200 and 350. This combination therapy is referred to as **"Highly Active Antiretroviral Therapy"** or **HAART** for short. This HAART combination of drugs **must** be taken every day for the rest of one's life. If treatment lapses, the virus then has an open window to develop resistance to the medications and all benefits up to that point will be lost. Taking two or more antiretroviral medications at the same time greatly reduces the rate at which drug resistance develops. http://www.avert.org/introtrt.htm.

So if you are on HAART **don't stop taking your meds !**

4. Only use clean sterile needles, and don't share needles. Boil the needle in briskly bubbling water for 20 minutes-if you must. That's how we did it in the OR back in the day to sterilize instruments before autoclaves!

Chapter 8

Death in the OR

Death in the operating room is a rare event, but it does happen. A lot depends on why you are having an operation, how sick you are to begin with and whether it is an emergent case or not. Trauma cases, such as car accident victims are unpredictable. There can always be surprises. Whenever a patient dies in the operating room, it is always the ultimate stressful event for everyone involved. The causes of death in the operating room vary. A patient's death in the operating room, whether under anesthesia or not, is usually associated to the underlying disease process as to why the patient is there in the first place. I've never witnessed a death in the OR where I worked due to an anesthetic issue. Nor did I ever witness a death in the OR due to a doctor's or nurse's fault.

For example, I was circulating nurse in a room where a car accident victim was being operated on to control bleeding. He was not conscious when he entered the OR room. He had multiple injuries to various internal organs. He had a punctured lung, a ruptured spleen, a lacerated liver and several fractures to one of his legs. The patient's spleen was removed as it is easier to remove it than to repair it, and besides, you can live without a spleen. I recall peeking into the surgical field before the skin incision was made. His abdomen looked normal. It did not look distended or disfigured in any way. There was no apparent bruising or any obvious lacerations. But when the surgeon made his lengthy midline incision parting the two abdominal muscles his internal injuries became apparent. Seeing beyond this gapping abdominal incision it was easily discernable to visualize the lethal fissures on his liver. The liver is ordinarily a smooth looking organ, but this patient's was not. There were these lacerations on his liver that were heavily pooled with bright red and partially clotted blood. As everyone knows, the liver is the largest organ in the human body weighing in between 1,200 and 1,600 grams or approximately 8 to 10 pounds of an adult's weight. Our livers are very vascular organs with huge arterial and venous blood supplies and it is important to note here that at any one given second a person's liver contains about 25% of an individual's circulating blood volume. This is a very critical fact regarding trauma victims. A person cannot live without a liver, so I knew we would be spending most of our time repairing this organ while simultaneously pumping units of both clotting factors (which is one of the liver's functions-producing clotting factors) and whole blood back into this patient. Since the adult human body contains approximately 10 pints of blood, I was sure I was looking at close to a pint of free uncirculating blood volume just sloshing about on top of his abdominal organs. Weighing bloody lap sponges and giving an accurate estimated blood loss (EBL) was going to be my most important responsibility for this patient. This EBL measurement would be documented and the surgeon and anesthesiologist would use my EBL measurement to replace blood products and other fluids. The patient's chart is a legal document and must be true and correct. No guessing allowed. The EBL must be measured and every bloody sponge weighed to the cubic centimeter. Likewise, the suction canisters have scored markings by the cc's and measuring and documenting this blood loss in these buckets must be frequently relayed to the anesthesiologist and surgeon as well. This young man's suction canisters immediately filled to the 400 cc mark as soon as the surgeon made his incision. I knew immediately this was going to be either a very long night, or a very short case depending on how this kid's heart held up. Youth was on his side.

Blood alcohol screening was performed on admission to the emergency room, and we received the report from the lab that the patient was legally intoxicated with a blood alcohol level of 2.1. The patient was actually thrown from the car as he was not wearing a seat belt either. That patient died as a result of his injuries. The surgeon documented on the patient's surgical post-op note that the cause of death was probably hypovolemic shock secondary to the blood loss due to the trauma of the car accident. In lay man's terms that means he literally bled to death. An individual will loose 20% of his circulating blood volume before developing hypovolemic shock. This patient probably was in hypovolemic shock upon entering the OR suite as I noticed he was tachycardic with a heart rate of 100 upon entering the room. Another clue was that he already had a unit of whole blood hanging on the

IV pole and infusing into his neck veins. The emergency room started replacing his blood volume before he arrived to us. He was loosing blood as fast as we were pumping it back into him. He was fighting to save his own life before we in the OR even touched him, as his heart was frantically trying to pump what little blood he had left through his arteries and into his vital organs. He was only 26 years old. He died. It was sad.

Lessons to be learned here are:
>   #1. Don't drink and drive
>   #2. Don't text and drive
>   #3. Always wear a seatbelt.

Utilizing either of these two good judgment decisions, buckling up and or not driving while intoxicated could have changed this young man's outcome drastically

When a patient dies in the OR it is truly a somber event. It never bothered me to take care of a deceased patient in the OR. I felt like even in death the patient still needed the nurses to care for him, his remains primarily to ease the families' suffering. When it would happen I would always imagine what the patient's family was doing and how upset they all must be. I would wonder how the surgeon would gingerly inform the family how everyone did all they could to save their loved one. However, there are certain rules and protocols that govern our nursing actions regarding the deceased patient. After all resuscitative measures have been exhausted and the patient is pronounced dead the surgeons and anesthesiologists will leave the operative suite and leave the deceased in the care of the OR nurses. The initial phase of post mortem care of patients who die in the OR begins with the OR nurses. It is imperative to note here that every patient who dies while in the operating room, especially while under anesthesia, automatically becomes a coroner's case and an autopsy most likely will be performed. All lines that have been placed into the patient, intravenous lines, and breathing tubes for example, and any other artificial portals must remain in place just as it was when it was inserted. It must not be tampered with in any way. I was told by an old friend who is a nurse anesthetist how another student anesthetist, upon initially intubating a paralyzed patient mistakenly placed the endotracheal tube (breathing tube) into the paralyzed anesthetized patient's esophagus. But the mistake was promptly discovered when the anesthetist's mentor/partner could not hear breath sounds over the patient's lungs via auscultation (listening with the stethoscope) while pumping oxygenated air into the endotracheal tube. He was ventilating the patient's stomach! Do not be alarmed because always in the OR whenever a patient is being anesthetized there are always two doctors who are anesthesiologists to assure that all goes smoothly, and sometimes three. If that scenario had been left uncorrected it would have taken less than 5 minutes for that patient to die. That would have been highly unlikely though, because after a few seconds, about 10 seconds, the anesthetized patient's heart rate would begin to escalate as the heart struggled to deliver freshly oxygenated blood, which there would be none because of the misplaced breathing tube. Additionally all the anesthetist's alarms would start alarming. Concurrently, the patient's pulse oxygen probe reading would start alarming as the oxygen saturation levels would drop from a normal 98% - 100% saturation rate to critical levels very rapidly. There are so many safeguards in the OR. The anesthesiologists I worked with at Jeff were perfectionists- they have to be! They were the best! I tell people they have a better chance of dying in a car accident on the way to the hospital than they do dying in the OR. Really !

The deceased patient's body is washed with water to remove all gross blood on the body's surface. Identification tags with the patient's name and medical record number are attached to the deceased. One tag is tied with a string to the patient's wrist and the other one around the big toe, just as depicted on the cover of the Mary Roach's bestselling book cover "STIFF" published in 2003. The patient's body is then placed in a white, body size, water impermeable bag. The bag is a soft white paper cloth material that will prevent any seepage of any body fluids from dripping onto anything. It folds around the patient like an envelope. There are no permanent closures like zippers or snaps. It's very clean looking. The only drainage I've ever witnessed in a deceased patient in the OR is urine leaking from a patient's bladder. Immediately when a person expires, all muscles in the body relax and become flaccid. Rigor Mortis, the stiffening of a corpse's muscles starts with the muscles of mastication (muscles used in chewing) and proceeds gradually descending from the head down to the muscles in the legs and feet. Rigor Mortis does not start until later (2-4) hours after death. Eventually the stiffening will subside in about 24 to 48 hours later and then the corpse's muscles will return to its flaccid state. Specialized circular muscles that constrict an opening or orifice called sphincters also relax. We human beings have nine sphincters scattered throughout our bodies performing specific functions. Most of them are in our digestive tracks. We have little or no control over their relaxing and contracting rhythms, except our urinary bladder's sphincter. Under normal circumstances, this urinary sphincter is constricted closing the orifice tightly. If it wasn't contracted or closed we'd be urinating and dripping urine almost constantly. On this particular deceased patient, her urinary bladder was not catheterized and we noticed as we turned her onto her side to wash her that the sheets under her bottom were soaked with urine.

Ordinarily, OR patients who die while in surgery have empty stomachs to begin with, as it is a pre operative order not to eat or drink 8 to 12 hours before surgery. The exceptions to this rule are emergency cases, like trauma patients who did not know they were going to crash their car into the telephone pole and have an emergency operation two hours after their cheese steak, or the teenager who drank a six pack of beer before hopping behind the steering wheel of his car. These people are usually intubated in the emergency room and any vomiting issues are attended to there. I've never seen anyone vomit during intubation in the OR in the more than 1,000 surgeries I participated. That's a pat on the back to the anesthesiology department and nursing personnel at my hospital, and that's the way it should always be, as the consequences to vomiting while under anesthesia, specifically immediately before and while being intubated can be morbid and lethal. Vomiting afterwards, now that's a different story. Everyone vomits in the RR or recovery room, but it's OK there because the paralyzing anesthetics given during the intubation process are worn off by the time you get to the recovery room, so you can control your airway and gag and cough and control your breathing. Believe me I've worked in the recovery room also, and having an emesis basin is standard operating equipment for each patient because EVERYONE VOMITS in the RR/PACU!

Upon death, peristaltic action or the normal bowel contractions cease. There is no seepage of stool from the large bowl after death, despite the relaxation of both the internal and external anal sphincters. Since there are no more rhythmic muscular contractions of the large bowel, neither stool contents or its gasses go anywhere. The bowels literally stop propelling and cave in on themselves. After death the bacteria that normally live in our bowels and that aid in the digestion of our food, will now flourish and multiply unchecked, as there is no longer a functioning immune system to regulate their numbers and these bacteria begin to eat and digest us instead. This bacterial action is not apparent to the observer's naked eye immediately after death, but it begins at the microscopic level, instantly and automatically upon our last breath. There is a "cadaver farm" located in the forests of North Carolina where the decay rates of cadavers are studied under various weathering circumstances and temperatures along with an entomologist's (studies insects) input and the results documented for reference to be used by whomever needs the information to determine time of death or other aspects of human decomposition. Police forensic departments and university forensic and anthropology students access this information frequently as it is utilized in the criminal justice arena, coroner's offices, medical schools and in the study of anthropology and forensics.

We can tell a lot about a person by looking into their eyes, especially if they're dead or not. Whether you know the person or not, looking into a dead person's eyes is truly a spooky event and something you never forget. My first patient who died in the OR was a man who expired after coronary bypass surgery. The first feature I noticed as I was washing his face was his eyes. Normally the anesthesiologist will tape the eyes shut for every procedure because while a person is anesthetized, frequently the patient will be paralyzed by some paralytic agent and without taping the eyelids shut the patient's eyelids will naturally fall open. While under anesthesia the patient cannot blink, produce tears, or keep his eyes shut, so we'll do it for him. After the patient expired after the surgical procedure, the anesthesiologist removed the thin white tape from his eyelids. His eyelids fell partially open. My fellow nurses who were with me during the case were busy doing other things. The scrub nurse was gathering the dirty surgical instruments and the shift charge nurse was on the telephone giving report to the floor as to the patient's death. It seemed as if I was all alone with this corpse. I started to gently wash his face and neck with cool water, then my curiosity got the better half of me. I leaned down, closer to the dead man's face. I got real close, as close as I could possibly get barring the endotracheal tube poking me in the nose. I lifted his right eyelid to a full circle. I immediately saw his lifelessness in my reflection in his dime sized pupil. His pupil was so large and dilated that it obscured all the color of his iris. I couldn't tell if he had blue, brown, hazel or even black colored eyes. I never peered so closely into a dead man's pupils before. I never had the opportunity. When I would go to the cadaver lab in the basement of the Medical College of Pennsylvania during nursing school as part of my anatomy and physiology class, all of the cadavers' eye balls were non existent as the vitreous humor, the clear jelly like fluid that occupies the orbit or globe as it is sometimes called, disintegrates rapidly after death. All of the cadavers' eye sockets were severely sunken in and all that remained in their places was what appeared to be flattened concave shaped dried prunes in what was once a round plump eyeball. I was used to checking pupillary reactions to light on patients' eyes in the SICU, on live patients as part of my nursing assessments, but those patients' pupils always reacted to light stimulation, even the unconsciousness ones, even if perhaps sluggishly. Only a brain dead person's eyes will not react to light. Whenever a light is shinned into one of your pupils, the pupil should constrict or get smaller and it should do so briskly, and when the light is taken away the pupil should dilate back to its starting normal size. And just as important, the reaction should be commensual; that is, when the light is shinned into one eye the reaction should be seen in both pupils equally, and at the same time. That's because our optic nerves crisscross in our brains, so in short, both our eyes share the same light sensations and, therefore both eyes should react identically to light regardless as to which eye is stimulated.

When we die, when our brains die, the ability of our eyes to sense light and react to light ceases, and so the muscles in our pupils stop constricting and they relax and dilate to the max, just like this man's did. Checking someone's pupillary reaction to light is a baseline assessment for determining if someone is brain dead. "Fixed and dilated" is the lingo used to describe a dead person's pupils. No reaction to light, no life. There are a very few circumstances where this does not happen, like if it's drug induced.

One of my favorite all time movies is Alfred Hitchcock's "Psycho". As great a film maker as Hitchcock was, I found a flaw in this classic thriller. As Janet Leigh lays prostate over the edge of a blood filled tub after being slashed to death by Anthony Perkins, AKA Norman Bates, the film maker has the cameraman zoom in for a close up of her dead face. The problem here is that her pupils are nearly pin point, and not dilated like a dead person's should be. Her small pupil size was most likely the result of normal pupillary constriction, a normal reaction to the camera lights being flashed directly into her eyes and face needed to film that shot. What would have made that scene more realistic is if a black contact lens colored to mimic a dilated pupil were used. Then she'd look really dead.

Many drugs can affect the size of one's pupils. The size of someone's pupil can also be indicative of drug abuse. People who abuse opium/heroin have smaller than normal pupils that don't dilate in the dark as they should. Heroin overdose patients have pinpoint pupils on admission the emergency room. Cocaine/crack/methamphetamine addicts - speed freaks display the opposite. They walk around with huge dilated pupils, during the daylight.

Sometimes we would perform surgery on brain dead people but not because anyone is trying to save their lives, but rather to save someone else's life. These people are organ donors. People who always die in the operating room are the potential organ donors who are brain dead to start. But not all organ donors are brain dead. For example there are thousands of live kidney donors. Many times family members, but mostly non relatives donate one of their kidneys to help others. People who sustain brain death the most are people who are stroke victims. But most brain dead organ donors are not stroke victims. The majority of brain dead organ donors are/were relatively healthy people who sustained a traumatic head injury, like motor vehicle and motorcycle accident victims, or victims of other traumatic events, perhaps a fall.

To be brain dead means to have irreversible cessation of all brain functions. Brain death occurs in trauma victims when the brain swells due to a traumatic injury. As the brain swells within the bony confines of the skull it expands to the point where the brain itself obstructs and cuts off its own oxygenated blood supply. The swelling literally strangulates the brain. Brain cells are very susceptible to lack of oxygen. It takes about 5 minutes without oxygen for brain cells to start dying. When brain cells start to decompose they liquefy. Any mortician will tell you that frequently the undertaker will have to plug the nasal cavity of a deceased person with cotton balls before a viewing because after 48 hours our brains will start draining through our noses. My father told me this. He went to mortuary school to become an undertaker, but he decided he couldn't do it and he became a barber instead.

There are certain criteria that the medical establishment uses to determine brain death before releasing a body for organ donation. It is a very complex and very legal matter. They just don't pull the plug. It sounds easy, but it isn't.

The first criteria is that the patient will be in a coma due to a known cause. Was the patient a car accident victim, or a head trauma victim? The cause of the coma must be known. You just can't use any dead person someone finds.

The second criteria demands that the patient will not have any brain stem reflex activity. These brain stem reflexes are involuntary reflexes. We have no conscious control over our brain stem reflexes. They are life sustaining reflexes and they are protective in nature. As anyone who has ever had a cough can attest to the fact that no matter how much Robitusin you take for that nagging cough, if you still have that post nasal drip draining into the back of your throat you're going to cough, and cough and cough no matter what. This is a defensive reflex our bodies use in order to clear our airways so we can breathe. The post nasal drip acts as a foreign body, so your cough reflex takes over to clear your airway. A brain dead person will not cough to clear his airway. A brain dead person will not have a **#1 cough reflex.** Another brain stem reflex that must be absent is the **#2 gag reflex**. Our gag reflex serves to maintain a patent airway also. If any foreign body attempts to enter the trachea/larynx and obstruct our breathing our gag reflex will work to expel and vomit out the obstruction. The brain dead patient will also have abnormal eye movements as related to head position, and nor will he blink. Just try not blinking the next time an eyelash falls into your eye! You'll have to blink because it's reflexive and you can't stop it. Thirdly, **#3**, our **corneal reflex** will react and close and blink the eyelid in order to protect the eye and to clear your eye so you can see, unless you're anesthetized, or brain dead. Also, the **#4 pupillary refex** to light in our eyes will be absent as well. If the patient's pupils in their eyes are fixed and dilated in response to light, they're brain dead. There's that term again, like that gentleman in the OR who died after his heart surgery. These are just a few examples. The

American Academy of Neurology has determined a check list of 25 criteria that must be met before a person can be pronounced brain dead (Neurology 2010; 74:1911-1978). I only explore a few here of what I used and saw and how they were used to assess for brain death.

Another very important criteria that is assessed is the patient's attempt to breath on his own when the respirator is disconnected. During this period of disconnection from the respirator, if a person's diaphragm does not contract to take in a breath, a person's CO_2 (carbon dioxide) level will rise as the oxygen level decreases and this will ultimately cause biological death. If the patient does not exhibit any spontaneous breathing after 10 minutes, he may be classified a brain dead. Rising CO_2 is the trigger that stimulates breathing. Breathing is automatic unless you are brain dead, or drugged. This is how a heroin overdose kills people. The narcotic opium suppresses respirations to the point where the blood's elevated CO_2 does not trigger the diaphragm to contract and signal the person breathe. This is what happens when we try to hold our breath as well. After 10 to 15 seconds the carbon dioxide level raises in our blood stream and we reflexively contract our diaphragm to suck in oxygenated air to breathe and to exhale or blow off excessive CO_2. We have to do it. We have no control over this autonomic reflex and the former brain stem reflexes, unless we're dead, and barring any paralytic agents, metabolic abnormality or hypothermia. We don't have to be conscious to do it either, just not brain dead. There are people who are in comas who are not brain dead and they breathe on their own for years. After all, we breathe all night long when we're asleep-an unconscious state. These are examples of what I as a RN did in assessing for brain death, and was involved with in assisting doctors when determining a patient's status for the possible preparation for organ donation. The full scope of testing for brain death is outside the scope of this book. The testing is very extensive and it must be accurate to insure that no mistake is made.

One donor patient whom I took care of in an ICU fits this sad scenario exactly. I had signed up to do a weekend of overtime with a local nursing agency, working at a hospital in the Kensington neighborhood of Philadelphia. It was the spring time of 1980. As I walked onto the ICU, I noticed two uniformed Philadelphia police officers sitting in chairs next to the entrance. I was assigned to care for a choking victim who had just been admitted to the ICU 2 hours before my arrival. He was in cubicle #4. He was a 24 year old, very thin male. During the patient report I asked, "What did he choke on?" I could see my patient from across the unit. His hands were tied to the railings of the bed and so were his feet. He had stopped having grand mal seizures by the time he arrived in the ICU. I though to myself at this point, "I'm gonna have my work cut out tonight."

"Well," said the reporting nurse, "This kid is a police matter. The police brought him in to the emergency room. He was a suspect in selling drugs, and when he was confronted by the police attempting to arrest him he swallowed the evidence, a bag of heroin. The bag of heroin subsequently became lodged and stuck in his throat. He started to choke. He couldn't swallow the evidence because the bag was too big to swallow. Plus it was in plastic wrap and that obstructed his airflow. Rumor has it that the police attempted to prevent him from swallowing the bag, the evidence, and a fight between the police and the patient ensued. The cops brought him here after he passed out from choking. He was having seizures in the ER but not any more. And now, here he is. He coded 3 or 4 times in the emergency room. He's now being evaluated for possible organ donation. They don't think he's going to make it. He might be brain dead," the reporting nurse told me. "The family is aware" she continued. I could see from 30 feet away that he had a tracheotomy and was attached to a ventilator as well. I thought to myself, "I better eat something now."

The entire night from 11 pm to 7 am I did nothing but take and assess my patient's vital life signs and assess for any brain stem activity/reflexes. Suctioning his tracheotomy to keep his airway patent took up most of my time. This young man ran the entire gamete of being prepared for organ donation. I worked the next evening too, because I got a bonus for working the entire weekend. This kid had undergone three EMGs, and a CAT scan of his brain over that 3 day weekend. My documentation was to be crucial in the assessment for brain death. I had to continually assess and document for any indications of brain stem activity, like breathing on his own or pupillary responses of which he had none. He was coughing a little when my shift started but by the end of the weekend he did not even cough when I suctioned his trach. He never responded to any painful stimulation, as he did not flinch when the skin on his arm was pinched. Nor did he ever attempt to breathe on his own when he was removed from the ventilator. His pupils in his eyes were sluggish to respond and were pretty dilated with each checking. When I left that ICU on 7 am that Monday morning, I had been informed that both of his kidneys were matched to recipients in the Philadelphia area and he would be undergoing bilateral nephrectomies (complete excision and removal of the kidneys and their veins and arteries) and the corneas of his eyes were to be removed later that day as well.

A CAT scan of the brain can also be utilized as criteria to assess for brain death. A CAT scan will confirm brain damage by visualizing any swelling of the brain due to trauma. And last but not least, an electroencephalogram (EEG) which measures brain electrical activity will be used to assess if the patient has any electrical brain activity. A flat EEG denotes no brain activity, and is used to verify brain death. Several EEGs over a time span of 3 to 5 days are the usual amount needed to confirm brain death. My patient's EEG revealed no brain activity.

And finally, if the patient who is classified as having brain death is a potential organ donor, that patient must be evaluated by two different physicians, neither of whom are the primary care givers of the potential organ recipient. Two physicians who are not associated with the organ recipient must be the people who will be responsible for the management, testing and certification of all procedures to be performed regarding any organ transplants. There must be no conflict of interest or bias. That would be unethical.

Examples of patients whom I knew were confirmed brain dead and their organs donated are many. Car accident victims, gun shot wound victims, fall victims, drowning victims, this choking victim, and a young healthy woman who was taking birth control pills and smoked cigarettes who threw a pulmonary embolism and stroked out, are examples of the donors I encountered in which I participated in the harvesting of their organs. The only comfort in seeing these young vibrant people pass is that they gave life, a better quality of life to others less fortunate. Most state motor vehicle agencies ask automobile drivers who are renewing their driving licenses if they want to be an organ donor in the case of a fatal accident, and the information is documented on their drivers' licenses. This tactic informs others, family members included that the licensed driver has made a conscious decision to donate his organs in this worst case scenario. This measure does not guarantee that his organs will be donated, but it raises awareness to the possibility.

The average healthy dead body, (an oxymoron, because how can one be dead and healthy at the same time?) can donate several organs. Two kidneys, one liver, one pancreas, bone marrow, one small intestine, two corneas, one heart, and two lungs and a bunch of tendons, ligaments, and skin are the organs transplantable today. Fourteen is the number I come up with. One donor can save the lives of 8 people and significantly improve the quality of life for 50 to 100 more. Is it worth it? In my opinion, Absolutely! The three year survival success rates for organ donation are as follows:

A. kidney donation is 95%
B. pancreas 92%
C. heart 91%
D. liver 90%
E. heart and lung 81%
F. 76% for lungs alone.

The US agency for Health Care Administration states that 13 people die daily waiting for donor organs. Our organs are useless to us when we are dead, as they'll only turn into human soup in a matter of hours to a few weeks, so why not ? It doesn't hurt. Just think of the joy, the happiness and the life that can be given to others; the child who needs a new heart, the sibling who needs a new kidney, and the cancer patient who needs the bone marrow. These stories are endless.

Just about everyone can become an organ donor. Even people with diabetes, cancer and some forms of hepatitis are acceptable. The only people who are excluded and who cannot become organ donors are people who test positive for HIV. There is a time window however, as to how much time can lapse between the time of death and the harvesting of the organ. These times vary according to the organ. Hearts and lungs must be harvested within six hours as these organs are very sensitive to lack of oxygen. The liver, pancreas and small intestines must be harvested within 24 hours, and the kidneys have a window of 48 hours. I signed my driver's license and checked off I want to be an organ donor in the case of a fatal car accident. My family is aware of my wishes.

While the organ donor is being evaluated for potential donation, he will be kept alive as if he were not brain dead. His blood gasses will be maintained at a normal oxygen saturation rate of 100%, his lung function will be normal with deep and adequate ventilation provided by a respirator, his heart rate will be monitored to assure normal function, and his kidneys will be properly hydrated as to maintain normal filtration and urine output. When we receive a donor patient in the operating room, as soon as the specified organ is harvested, or removed from the body, the incision is closed. No dressings need to be applied. The respirator is turned off. Then the operating room staff waits for approximately 3 to 5 minutes for the donor's heart rate to flat line, if not being harvested itself. At that moment the donor patient is not only brain dead, he is now officially clinically and biologically dead. The time of death is documented on the chart. The nurses commence to care for the donor patient like others who have died in the OR. The washing and tagging of the body is performed, and then the body is taken by gurney to the hospital morgue or pathology lab, or to the funeral parlor.

All patients who expire in the operating room, including some donor patients will automatically become coroner's case and will undergo an autopsy. However, the coroner has the authority to decide how extensive the autopsy should be. He or she will determine whether to perform a complete autopsy, which includes opening the skull and examining the brain, or to perform a limited autopsy, or a selective autopsy. A limited autopsy examines the deceased person's body from the neck down, excluding the head and brain. The third type of autopsy is a selective autopsy. This third type of autopsy examines only a specific body system or organ. This type of autopsy might be done to confirm a specific disease that the deceased most likely had. An example would be to examine a person's liver to determine how extensive his hepatitis was and if he really had cirrhosis or cancer in addition as a co-morbidity factor. Another example of a selective autopsy would be a gunshot victim. The coroner might only examine the cavity in which the bullet entered the body and will document the extent of damage done to specific organs or vessels so to correctly document the cause of death.

People who expire and have a fever of unknown origin are also mandated to have an autopsy. These people might be carrying potentially lethal communicable diseases like bacterial meningitis, Jacob-Creutzfeldt disease, otherwise known as Mad Cow disease, hepatitis of any variety, B, C, or D, HIV, or whatever other mysterious infectious disease that needs to be reported to the CDC. Likewise, the operating room nurse who is in charge of tagging the body before transport to the morgue must also identify with a toe tag that the body is to be handled with "Infection Precautions" and the suspected organism stated so as to communicate to the pathologist and fellow co-workers who will be handling infectious bodily liquids or organs. All autopsies usually include taking cultures from various tissues, as well as blood cultures, to confirm whether or not the deceased carried any infectious diseases and if that specific organism contributed to the cause of death.

Deaths occurring within one week of an invasive procedure are mandated for autopsy as well. These procedures include but are not limited to angioplasty, chest tube insertion, induced abortion, and central line insertion. I have a neighbor who underwent an angioplasty of one of his coronary arteries for a stent insertion. One week later he started slurring his words and developed blindness in one of his eyes. Upon admission to the hospital it was discovered that the tip of the inserted line broke off, and acting as a clot, the tip traveled through his blood stream and lodged into the tiny vessels in his brain and he had a stroke. He survived the stroke and is much better today, but not 100%. This scenario could have been disastrous and it could have killed him.

A woman who dies within twenty weeks of an induced abortion will also become a coroner's case. Infections and pulmonary emboli (blood clot in the lung) will be suspect regarding this scenario.

After the nurses are finished preparing the body, the nursing assistant will take the deceased's body to the morgue in the hospital.

All autopsies are performed by a forensic pathologist. The forensic pathologist is a MD or a DO who furthers his studies in forensics. "Quincy" the television coroner was a forensic pathologist and so is "Dr. G. Medical Examiner". She is good. I just love her TV show. Only a forensic pathologist or the medical examiner (ME) has the authority to state the "manner of death" as well as the cause of death. The ME will also use information on the patient's chart in determining co-factors to the cause of the deceased's death. These two terms "Manner of death" and "cause of death" sound alike but they are not. Manner of death pertains to the legal determination of circumstances surrounding the death of the deceased. The medical examiner can state the manner of death using one of five terms:

A. Natural
B. Homicide
C. Suicide
D. Accidental
E. or undetermined

A perfect example of the difference between the two terms is the death of a person who died as a result of falling off a horse. His manner of death is documented as "Accidental", yet the cause of death was an infection or septicemia. This person sustained an accidental fall from his horse. The fall fractured his spine and left him paralyzed from the neck down. Subsequently, his immobility due to his paralysis left him with deep pressure sores on his body. Those sores became infected and the infection ran rampant through his body. He became septic and died of "Septicemia" or an infection was the cause of death, but "Accidental" was the manner of death- or the circumstance that set up the cascading events that portended his septicemia and death. Obviously his manner of death was not homicide, or suicide, or natural, or unknown.

CHAPTER 9

MY WIFE NEEDS A NEW MINK COAT

Over time, as my career as an operating room nurse progressed, I noticed that the hospital started hiring more OR techs to act as first assistant scrub nurses. These OR techs went to specialized schools to learn this highly skilled job, and they were a welcome asset to the OR staff. Their expertise in anatomy was solid. Being able to hire a trained professional that can start work immediately without extensive on the job training is valuable to any employer. This meant that the RNs were utilized increasingly as the circulating nurse component of the OR team, only now almost exclusively. As usual there is always nursing shortage. I'm sure this fact was the catapulting factor in this administrative decision, to go with OR surgical techs. State laws ubiquitously have always mandated that only a RN could circulate anyway, she just didn't have the luxury of scrubbing perhaps, as much as she wanted. The RN was in a sense the manager of the room. This function required detail to documentation on the patient's chart because as stated before, the patient's chart is a legal document. Only licensed professionals like doctors, surgeons, nurses, or physical therapists and other health care professionals are privy to documenting unbiased scientific facts on it. It has to be exact.

I always liked scrubbing for cases because it was never boring. Every patient was different and unique, and every procedure had its individual twists and surprises. I always took the opportunity to scrub rather than circulate, because being the circulating nurse can at times be dull and mundane, but when I scrubbed my day seemed to flash by. On this particular day I was working the relief shift, 10am to 6pm. I didn't have an assigned room. I floated from room to room relieving both circulating and scrub nurses for lunch breaks, and when 3pm rolled around, I would relieve that nurse for the day and continue with that case until it finished or 6pm, my time to split. At 3pm I entered a mastectomy case as the relieving scrub nurse. I knew I would be assigned to that case for the remainder of the day because the case was just starting. I could see the surgeon making the skin incision on the patient through the door window. I wasn't exactly happy to be assisting with this particular surgeon because he was known to be a little snappy. He was one of those people who was overly critical of everything from the temperature in the room to the radio station I selected. I donned the sterile gown and gloves and the case started without delay. This particular patient, a middle aged woman was having a right mastectomy for breast cancer. The surgical team numbered four. It was the attending surgeon, two male surgical residents and me at the field. Since the hospital where I worked was a teaching university hospital, every OR case was a teaching instruction as well. The OR cases provided surgical education and experience for the surgical residents. Hey, it was a medical college! The surgeon let all of us palpate the woman's breast tumor, one at a time so we could have the opportunity of experiencing what a cancerous tumor felt like. The patient's right breast was still attached to her torso. It had been 15 minutes since the initial skin incision, but a sizable area the breast was already dissected. Her right breast kind of hung open like a door hinged to her armpit. The tumor was ensconced within thick layers of adipose (fat) tissue. Without seeing the patient before she entered the OR, and even though she was completely covered by surgical drapes, it was evident to me that she was an obese woman.

The tumor was irregular in shape, about the size of a golf ball, and cement rock hard. It was harder than hard if that's possible. It had a density all its own. The mass had a gritty spike like almost sharp edge that could be felt beneath its thick layer of adipose tissue. It had to have been growing for years. I thought to myself 'Clearly this patient was not a candidate for a lumpectomy because her tumor was so large.' Encountering situations like this makes you acutely aware of your own mortality. As a woman, to me it was very scary. I tried not to let the others know that it bothered me, but it was definitely anxiety producing. I promised myself that if I ever knew or suspected that I had a breast lump that I would not let it go to this point. To this day I check my breasts for lumps 2 to 3 times a week. Seeing and knowing the worst makes me worry too much! Too much knowledge skews my perception of reality.

The conversation in the room turned to the latest movie blockbuster "Back to the Future". The surgeons and

I laughed and took turns telling our favorite funny parts of the movie. I stood immediately to the right arm of the attending surgeon. He continued to skillfully carve off the patient's cancerous right breast with a cauterizing knife. The use of a cautery blade instead of a scalpel for this surgery controls bleeding readily and makes the procedure go rather quickly instead of clamping and tying off of each tiny bleeder. I balanced a sterile 1,000 ml stainless steel specimen bowl atop the patient's abdomen awaiting the reception of the cancerous breast. I did not want to chance handling the specimen with my hands because the breast tissue was so large and gelatinous, and I did not want to drop it on the floor. The aroma of burning human flesh and hemoglobin permeated the air. Circles of smoke from the cautery blade choked my nostrils with the stench of charred human flesh, despite wearing a surgical mask that covered my nose and mouth. The smell of human tissue burning is like nothing I've ever smelled before working in the operating room. It's a smell you never forget. It smells like metal, as the iron or hemoglobin in our blood is cooking and is on fire. It was a very distinctive smell and I could never get used to it. It's different from other animals and this how I know.

I believe all animals have their own scent. Case in point: While I was working for a visiting nurse home care agency, I once had a patient whom I visited who had a very unusual pet. When I entered his home I first observed how meticulously it was decorated with delicate antiques. Every table, every shelf was covered with fine pieces of colored glass and dainty nick knacks. I gingerly navigated my way through his home, so as not to bump into anything with my bulky nursing bag. I also noticed that the home had a sweet home cooking kind of smell to it, like country smoked bacon. They must have had breakfast just before I entered. As I was sitting beside my patient to take his vital signs, something caught my peripheral vision from within the adjoining room. A huge 500 lb., 5 ft. long fat brown pig waddled from across the living room to greet me. I nearly fainted. I wanted to scream, but my patient started chuckling and reassured me that "Molly" was his pet and she would not hurt me. Molly stuck her porky nose up against my legs and started sniffing me, then she waddled away obeying her master's commands to "Go sit", which she did, just like a dog. I was afraid "Molly" was going to take a bite out of my calf, but she didn't. My patient told me that Molly, and pigs in general are very intelligent animals. My patient also told me how pigs are very loving and obedient animals. He explained how pigs were smarter than dogs and how they are very easy to house train. He continued to explain how "Molly" was the best pet he ever owned. I was amazed! Who knew?!!!! I wouldn't have believed it if I hadn't seen it with my own eyes! Enough of my pork encounter, but this serves to demonstrate the distinctiveness between animal smells. Human flesh has its own aroma just like Molly the pig's house smelled like delicious smoked bacon! How cool! Molly had left her mark, her BO scent. People laugh today when I tell this story and how funny it is because it is so true! I shun eating pork because I know this animal "Molly" is a being who I believe truly has a loving soul. Back to the OR:

It takes about forty five minutes to an hour to do a mastectomy. We were almost done the bulk of the procedure as the patient's breast was just hanging by threads of fatty tissue and a flap of skin. I repositioned the specimen pan close to the surgeon's hands so he could easily place it into the sterile container. As he was cauterizing the last attachments of flesh from between her torso and her breast when that insensitive surgeon said to his unconscious, anesthetized, completely unaware patient, the woman whose insurance company was going to pay him thousands of dollars, said in his self righteous condescending tone of voice, "Come on lady, my wife needs a new mink coat" ! I immediately looked over to the senior resident to visually confirm I heard what I thought I heard. I couldn't believe it! I didn't think what he said was funny. The resident gave me a quick glance, closed his eyes for one second and shook his head, oh so subtly in disbelief. I knew this attending surgeon was at times obnoxious, but this statement was completely uncalled for. It was disrespectful at the very least to me, because I was fully conscious and awake, and he knew I heard him, but to say that to a sick woman, behind her back and unknowing with cancer, a potential terminal disease, was nauseating. At that moment in time, I realized that this guy didn't really give a shit about this poor woman's plight. In my opinion, he only was caring about himself. I wondered if all he actually was calculating was how much money he would make by cutting off her breast. He should not have jokingly made that remark, especially in front of other people. If he thought he was funny, he wasn't. Clearly he was helping this woman to cure her disease, but somewhere in my heart I didn't believe it. He was in a position of power. He called the shots. The surgeon is the "captain of the ship" in the OR. No one responded to his snide remark. Not even me. Everyone remained silent. What could anyone possibly say in response to such a callous remark? Perhaps, "Oh, What color of mink does your wife like better, black or white" or maybe "Does she prefer a stole or a jacket?" I should have gone to my supervisor but I was afraid to do so. If I did report him, then he would know who reported him and I would have to come to work fearful of retaliation. So I did nothing. I felt intimidated because I knew this man could be very arrogant and domineering, especially if anyone angered him. I did not want to be the person to piss him off. I might loose my job if I spoke up. I needed my job.

This was the second time of several instances in my nursing career that a physician, a man of authority exposed his self righteousness, his opulence, his arrogance and his insensitivity toward me and or women. From then on, I always questioned some male physicians' motives. I would ponder if doctors really cared about their patients, or did they only enter the profession because it would make them rich. I never saw a poor doctor. I don't want to believe that all doctors are vainglorious, but let reality speak. Frequently, almost daily I would see the doctors I knew from the OR at the parking garage. They all drove the latest models of Mercedes, Corvettes, Jaguars and Porches. So did I, but there's more to it. But doctors work hard, and in order to be a physician you have to be very smart, bright, sincere and very dedicated. 99% of the physicians I know and worked with fit this mold. Like a lightning bolt, an idea flashed in my mind. One very huge chunk of realization regarding my profession became white diamond clear. Nurses are not independent in their own right, because they are women (my opinion). Nurses always work for other people, making other people profitable, (hospitals and businesses, and health care institutions) and their administrators are paid heftily. RNs are paid at the bottom of the heap. Nurses very often work for doctors and hospitals, and are dependent on them for their livelihoods. Nurses cannot bill for their services independently to an insurance company or charge a patient out right for their performance or skills. Like, I could not charge that breast cancer patient whom I cared for in the OR, scrubbed for and assisted the surgeon during the operative procedure for my OR nursing surgical expertise. But the doctor can. I am a licensed health care professional too, just like the doctor, only my nursing services are viewed differently on a monetary scale. The nursing profession is predicated on "taking orders." I call the profession of nursing

"The Profession of Oppression", because not only are nurses/women degraded by male doctors, other authority figures, and healthcare institutions alike, but they are also degraded and victims of lateral violence by their peers and coworkers, by other registered nurses as well. 20 % of new RNs leave the nursing profession altogether during the first 2 years due to

"Lateral Violence" inflicted on them by fellow RNs (http://ccn.aacnjournals.org/content/27/3/10). That's another book in the making. "Despite how many degrees a nurse obtains, a baccalaureate, a masters or even a PhD, or how hardworking and how smart nurses are, or how they bust their asses on the night shift, in the ER, the OR, the DR, or the ICU, saving life, after life, after life, or how much independence they think the profession awards them, you'll never see a rich nurse, unless she's married to a doctor, or leaves the profession for another. That's my opinion.

CHAPTER 10

ABORTION

It's the law. On January 22, 1973 the Roe vs. Wade decision allowing abortion was handed down by the US Supreme Court and it became legal to obtain an abortion. Whether to have an abortion or not is a tough decision for any woman to make. I do not claim allegiance to either cause, Pro-life or Pro-choice. I only wish to communicate the reality of both sides to all women based on my personal professional operating room nursing woman's point of view. Most people have not witnessed the actual procedure, held a dead fetus or embryo or products of conception in their hands, nor dealt with the emotional and psychological consequences that women who've had an abortion have endured, like I have witnessed regarding this issue. I cared for hundreds, maybe thousands of women in the pre-OR, the operating room itself, delivery room, and recovery room who made the decision to take this controversial course of action. The decision is never black or white.

Surprisingly, having an abortion is way more common than you can imagine. Worldwide, there are approximately 46 million abortions performed per year. Yes, I said **46,000,000** abortions per year. That reduces to approximately 126,000 abortions per day. Whoa! I had no idea of this until I did the research for this book. Here in the United States, there are approximately 1.37 million abortions performed yearly and 3,700 done per day. Planned Parenthood estimates that the worldwide lifetime average is about 1 abortion per woman on the planet. The reasons for having an abortion are varied. It is documented by sources obtained from Planned Parenthood that rape and incest account for a surprisingly **less than 1 %.** Only 6 % attribute health reasons of the mother or the fetus. Most women, 93% state that the reason for their decision to abort was that their pregnancy was not planned and either she or her partner desired to terminate the pregnancy. These statistics are what I've researched and are clearly documented in various professional journals. But being as curious as I am/was, I took it a step further. Consequently, I've spoken to hundreds of women, maybe thousands while I was working the GYN wing of the operating room and I found that their reasons were exactly the same as those published by statistical researchers. The big difference is that I saw the personal side of those huge numbers. The decision to have an abortion is not an easy one. The women I encountered were all very emotional regarding their decisions. Some were angry. Most were sad. Many verbalized freely. Others were dead quiet and couldn't wait till it was over. Some refused to look me in the eye when I spoke to them. They would look away and stare at some distant object. A few cried. None were happy, in my opinion. I never saw any smiles. I can't believe I had the nerve to do what I did, but I had to know. I asked so many of these women, "Why?" "What made you make the decision to have an abortion?" All of these women seemed to need to talk; perhaps looking or reaching for approval. Or were they grieving? They were all in need of comfort or of reassurance. I supported all of their decisions and verbalized to each of them that "I understood" even if I really didn't. That was my job. Injecting guilt into someone's soul is a cruel thing to do because no one ever knows what really goes on behind closed doors and no one, especially me, a health care professional should ever judge. They don't teach 'mind reading' in nursing school. If there is any point I need to emphasize and communicate regarding this issue, it is to "NEVER JUDGE!" No matter how much you think you know, believe me you don't. I wondered what their thoughts were. "Is this the right decision? It's too late now! I'm here!" might be one thought. All of their stories were different. I believe that they were all hurting and in need of healing, but not necessarily a physical healing but rather an emotional purge.

Here is a sampling of some of the reasons women told me why they chose abortion. They are as follows:

1. I'm married and it's my boyfriend's baby. My husband doesn't know.

2. I'm not married and it's my brother-in-law's baby, my sister's husband. No one knows.

3. Most of the women were unmarried. I didn't count, but I know they were. According to Planned Parenthood, 64.6 % of women seeking abortions are unmarried.

4. My baby has trisomy 13, Downs Syndrome.

5. My baby has trisomy 11, Downs Syndrome.

6. My baby has a heart defect.

7. My baby's brain did not develop.

8. A young lady had been in a car accident and had multiple leg and hip fractures. She had greater than 30 x-rays to her pelvic area and she never knew she was pregnant. I remember she was very upset and she was crying while she waited her "TURN."

9. A high class middle aged mother with a kick ass manicure escorted her teary eyed 16 year old teenage daughter to the OR. The first words out of this mother's mouth to me were, "She's not having this "THING." I just bit my tongue.

10. I can't afford it.

11. I'm still in college. 64.4 % of all abortions are performed on never married single women, and 52 % of women obtaining abortions are younger then 25 years old. http://www.abortionno.org/Resources/fastfacts.html.

12. "My parents will be so angry with me. How can I face my family? I'm Catholic." 31% of aborting women claim to be Catholic. (The Alan Guttmacher Institute, 1998, www.agi-usa.org.) Jewish women account for 1.8 % of abortions.

13. Caucasian women receive 60% of all abortions. African American women are 3 times as likely to have an abortion, and Hispanic women are 2 times as likely as white women to obtain an abortion http://www.abortionno.org/Resources/fastfacts. html/. Most of the women I saw having abortions were Caucasian.

Regardless of the reason, these women were in need of care, both physical care and emotional and psychological care. That was my job as a nurse; to care for my patients without judgment. To have an abortion can be a life altering decision. Some are stoic and view the event as just another necessary medical procedure, but some women find out later that they are not capable of carrying the emotional baggage. There are significant emotional and psychological consequences regarding a woman's decision to abort. For most women who have had abortions, their decision was the best for them at that time and they report no deleterious emotional or psychological after effects. Every woman's capacity to juggle the emotional consequences associated with abortion is different. However, in an article published by the British Journal of OB & GYN researchers identified that 31 % of women had regretted having their abortions. We don't hear about this phenomenon in the news. We don't read about this in "TEEN" or "GLAMOUR" magazines either. But it exists. Roe vs. Wade was good for some, but not psychologically or emotionally healthy for all. I've seen the sadness on theses girls' faces. For that minority of women who regret aborting their children, and 31% is a big minority, I believe that abortion is an act of desperation that may haunt them the rest of their lives. An abortion does not cure a disease, nor does it provide healing of any condition or correct a problem, or heal a relationship of any kind. Pregnancy is a normal healthy state of being. The evidence lies in the fact that there are thousands of medical practices in the USA that specialize in infertility or trying to make women achieve a pregnancy who otherwise cannot, because of various endocrine or other impacting diseases. Professionally speaking, outside of legal medical circumstances, I believe that the reality is that it is the negative social stigma surrounding an unplanned pregnancy that needs to be fixed, cured or corrected, not the pregnancy itself, because rushing off to abort a healthy baby is not going to fix any social problem. When abortion first became accepted as an ethical alternative, many people rejoiced because their **choice** was now "Legal", and it was no longer a sin or a crime to have an abortion. But now we have a new set of problems related to our new found freedom of choice. It is a fact, that since abortion's legalization the literature is filled with documentation stating the negative after effects of abortion. Stories abound on how abortion has created a new set of problems affecting a woman's' emotional and psychological health; Specifically, guilt, depression, anger, nightmares, suicide, and anxiety disorders now occur in a large numbers of these women, who before their abortion did not have. In my opinion there are times when an abortion can cause more distress in the long run because we are thinking short term regarding the immediate circumstance, and we are not thinking long term, and of the entire health of the woman over her life span, encompassing future physical, psychological and mental well being. And I'm a democrat! I feel the need to bring this issue forward, thereby arming women, young and old, mothers and sisters, daughters and cousins alike with information regarding this negative entity. These detrimental consequences regarding abortion are what needs addressing and be made known before a woman decides. I don't care who is right and who is wrong, Pro-life or Pro-choice, we all need to step back and look at the problems the decision of Roe vs. Wade has created for this significant minority portion of women who choose to abort. It took years for us to realize that abortion is not a quick fix for an undesired social situation. Suicide, especially in teenagers, emotional disorders, anxiety disorders, sleep disturbances and increased usage of prescribed psychotropic medications have all been documented in the literature for years as the most health altering events after an induced abortion. A new psychological phenomena has been named and it is called **"Post Abortion Squeal."** http://www.afterabortion.org/2006/. Its incidence and prevalence has been documented since the early 1970's when abortion entered mainstream legal medicine. The less support the woman has regarding her decision to terminate a pregnancy, the higher the incidence of this negative event. Single women (64%), divorced women, and teenagers fall into this increased risk category for the development of Post Abortion Squeal. This "Post Abortion Squeal" or **"PAS"** is a form of **"Post Traumatic Stress Disorder" (PTSD),** like the post- traumatic stress disorder soldiers sometimes develops after war/combat. When the stressor or traumatic event is an abortion, **PAS** is the term used to pinpoint the specific event causing the post traumatic stress disorder (PTSD).

Post Traumatic Stress Disorder (PTSD) has been documented by Hermann/Stewart (1992), to occur in approximately 19% of women post abortion. PTSD can be defined as a psychological dysfunction occurring after a traumatic experience, physical, emotional, or psychological which overwhelms an individual's normal defense mechanisms. According to the Diagnostic and Statistical Manual of Mental Disorders (DSM-4) this PTSD results after the onset of a traumatic experience that compromises the physical integrity of its victim. Many women may interpret and associate an abortion as a traumatic event. In a book titled "Forbidden Grief: The Unspoken Pain of Abortion by Theresa Burke with David Reardon (Acorn Books, 2002), Ms. Burke writes how some women describe their abortions like being "surgically raped." Coercion from family members, a boyfriend, lover, other friends, or by a parent who may try to persuade a woman into having an unwanted abortion is common. But no one really knows how common that practice is, because no one ever admits to pressuring anyone into having an abortion. There are no statistics to document its prevalence. Or at least I could not find any. The incidence of duress and its correlation to abortion is/or has never been measured or had a quantatative number given to it. This domineering pressure by significant others can leave the woman feeling helpless and out of control. A woman having an abortion under duress may also experience feelings of intense fear, or a feeling of being trapped and having no choice. So much for Pro-Choice! All too often, women will seek abortion because of a domineering or controlling figure because these outside people want the abortion more than the women does. This is anecdotal evidence as there are no statistics on how many abortions are forced upon women. Who is going to admit to that???? The realities are not revealed until after the fact when the problems associated with PAS arise. These domineering other people will state that they want what is good for the woman or what is best for the woman, but they are actually imposing their own selfish desires and placing their own needs ahead of the woman's and the unseen unborn child's true needs. That's my opinion. It could be a boyfriend who doesn't want to enter into a long term commitment, like marriage with the girl and/or who doesn't want the obligation of decades worth of child support payments. Or perhaps it's the parents who are convincing their teenage daughter that her life will be better without the obligations she would endure as a single parent. Or maybe the father is already married to someone else and for whatever reason he doesn't want anyone to know. Who knows? The woman may feel violated by these significant others and be pressured into making the "right decision". I'll never forget a scenario mimicking this statement's scenario.

While I was working in the reception area of the gynecological operating room where the abortions were performed, a somber 16 year old girl entered. She was so pretty she could have been a fashion model. Her mother followed closely behind her stretcher. I knew she was 16 years old because of the DOB stamped onto her wrist ID band. She had just had a birthday the month before. As I started to ask the teenage patient some routine questions, her mother abruptly interjected, "My daughter is not going to have this **"THING"**. I knew what she meant. I did not respond. I acted as if I did not hear her, but I knew she knew I did. I looked down at the adolescent and noticed that her eyes were teary, and her bottom lip was quivering. She had been crying. Why, I could only guess. I thought that maybe she was crying because she was having an abortion that she really did not want to have. ??? Or was she crying because she missed her boyfriend? Or was she crying because she really wanted this baby? Or, was the teen being coerced into having the abortion, because obviously her mother really wanted the abortion??!!! This was a very touchy situation. I wondered was the teenager the legal consent giver, or was the mother pulling all the strings? All I was sure of was that this was not the place, nor the time for family counseling, especially by me. All of the paper work was in order. The 16 year old was the person who signed the consent. She had her abortion.

But I recognized that this child was obviously experiencing a depressive episode. This kid was scared to death, and I could not do squat! Clearly, she would be a candidate for developing PAS. I could only pray that she would receive some kind of help or therapy afterwards, to help her deal with her superimposed grief, guilt, and depression. This exact patient is the reason why I believe that there should be counseling before any abortion. I also believe that the counseling be private to assure that the woman is not being forced or coerced into having the abortion and to assert also that it is her "Choice" and not someone else's, especially in the case of adolescents.

During my research I learned the symptoms of PAS/PTSD and I want to share these with anyone and everyone experiencing this similar situation so you could recognize the red flags and seek counseling. PAS is exhibited in three primary ways according to Speckhard, 1987,Rue, V.

& Speckhard, A. (1992a). Informed consent & abortion: Issues in medicine and counseling. Medicine and Mind 6 (1-2) (pg. 75-94). (1987). Hyper arousal behaviors are common. This behavior is depicted as constantly having a "turned-on" or chronically aroused "fight or flight" defense mechanism. Symptoms might include insomnia, anxiety attacks, or irritability. Another behavior may be "Intrusion reactions." This means the woman may experience the memory of the traumatic event over and over again at unexpected and undesirable times. The thought of the abortion intrudes upon and or interrupts her daily routine. It is always popping up in her mind. An example of this may be the woman having little flashbacks of the event or having anniversary reactions, where as she might experience surging feelings of guilt or depression on or around the aborted baby's due date and it's expected birthday, or on the anniversary of the abortion. That date will always have a black cloud over it. Watching diaper commercials on television or seeing children playing in a playground can become unbearable.

Another way that PAS/ PTSD may be exhibited is what is known a "constriction" or avoidance behavior. Here the woman will try to deny or avoid the negative feelings associated with the abortion. She might withdraw from relationships with people associated with and who knew about the abortion, and those who impacted her decision to have the abortion. She might also avoid contact with children altogether. She might hold back or suppress any tender or loving feelings toward others. She may withdraw from previously joyous activities. She may ultimately just emotionally shut down. Ms. Burke in her book describes this avoidance behavior in a client who had an abortion and associated running the vacuum cleaner in her home with the abortion procedure as she remembered the sound of the suction machine used during her abortion, as it is a vacuum that sucks out the products of conception right out of one's uterus. Self-destructive thoughts or suicide may invade her mind (Speckhard, Psycho-social Stress Following Abortion, Sheed & Ward, Kansas City: MO, 1987; Gissler, Hemminki & Lonnqvist, "Suicides after pregnancy in Finland, 1987-94: register linkage study," British Journal of Medicine 313:1431-4).

An article in the British Journal of Medicine (1996) by Haignare, et, al, reports a suicide ideation rate of 60% in those women who experienced PAS. Alarmingly, 28 % of post abortion women actually attempted suicide, and of these, half attempted suicide twice. Sadly, suicide attempts are significantly more prevalent among teenage post abortion women. Adolescent women may feel the most alone as they do not have the familial support of their loved ones. The teenager may not be married and may not have a significant other partner, or the parents might reject the pregnancy and offer no support. Teenagers also lack the emotional and social maturity to handle such adult situations and feel they have nowhere to turn. Teenagers may be ridiculed or bullied by their peers, as we all remember high school can be so very cruel. At a time in their lives when an intact self esteem is important, and social issues weigh heavily upon one's self worth, the pregnant teenager may feel like her life is imploding, that she is all alone and there is no hope, no way out. Likewise, teenagers may have the least support from their boyfriends as they may be adolescents themselves, and are not emotionally secure themselves and not financially able to support offspring at that time. Teenagers may feel more ashamed and embarrassed by an illegitimate pregnancy, and some may experience and will succumb to outside social pressures and experiment with alcohol or other substance abuse. A teenager might be subject to judgment by classmates or other adults, perhaps even teachers. Subsequently, the teenager may develop lowered self-esteem and be prone to engaging in risky behaviors, which are associated with PTSD and PAS. I know of a high school girl in the next town over from me who committed suicide over an unplanned pregnancy. She hung herself in her bedroom closet. She was a high school junior.

If you are a woman who is pregnant and your boyfriend says he'll leave you if you carry through with the pregnancy, believe me, he already has plans to leave you anyway. This type of man is a manipulator and is only thinking of his own needs. A man who threatens you with ultimatums doesn't love you, so drop him. Love is not conditional. The suicide rate for women 1 year post abortion is 6 times greater than for women who gave birth at term according to a Scandinavian study published in the British Journal of Medicine in 1996(18 Gissler M, Hemminki E and Lonnqvist J. Suicides after pregnancy in Finland, 1987-94: register linkage study. British Medical Journal 1996 December 7;313(7070):1431-4).

Sexual dysfunction is also an unfortunate squeal to induced abortion. Skeckhard (1987) reports a 30% to 50% incidence of sexual dysfunction in post abortion women. Dysfunctional sexual behaviors include loss of pleasure with inability to reach orgasm, increased vaginal pain with intercourse, and / or complete aversion to sex with men. This onset of sexual dysfunction occurs immediately after abortion.

Unfortunately, as with any surgical procedure, there are physical complications associated with induced abortion. These are rarely publicized. In an article published in 2004 in the American Journal of Obstetrics and Gynecology, the authors reported that the death rate associated with abortion is 2.95 times higher than that associated with pregnancies carried to term (40 weeks gestation). Surprisingly, women who were pregnant and carried to term had the lowest mortality (death) rate than ever non-pregnant women. According to the CDC (2005), complications of legal abortion are documented as the 5th leading cause of death in women of childbearing age. The most common causes of death in women post abortion are in order of frequency:

1. Hemorrhage
2. Infection
3. Pulmonary embolism
4. Anesthesia death
5. Undiagnosed ectopic pregnancy

For more information regarding these statistics log onto www.afterbortion.org.

I never saw a death of a woman due to abortion in the operating room or the recovery room in the 10 years I worked there. The only complication I saw was one time, a repeat of the procedure for bleeding because of retained POC (products of conception). But death due to induced abortion will not occur in the operating room that day, rather the above stated causes of death happen hours, weeks, and sometimes months later. A post abortion death may very well be missed, as the woman might present ill weeks or months later with a complication and it not be attributed to the abortion weeks before, as the patient may not disclose her history, or if the woman presents **DOA – dead on arrival** at the hospital. There is no way of knowing.

Abortion is done in several ways. The usual method performed is by suction. This method is usually done in the first trimester, and is easy and quick. There is the morning after pill too, which is really not an abortion, rather it is just a prevention measure so the embryo cannot implant into the uterine wall, if conceptions even occurred at all. That's not really an abortion. Also, one might not ever really conceive, so you actually never know if you were pregnant or not by using the morning after pill.

The age of the fetus also determines the method. If the fetus is in the 2nd or 3rd trimester it is more difficult as the baby is literally killed in the womb and cut up into pieces so it can be easily removed through the cervix. Some body parts will not fit into and through the suction tubing. This type of abortion is rare, and many times illegal. In the early 1970's while in nursing school I was introduced to the care of women who were undergoing the saline abortion method. It was the first time I ever witnessed an abortion of any kind. I was a nursing student, an 18-19 year old teenager myself when I was assigned to a patient having a "Saline abortion."

Saline abortions were the type utilized in a 2nd trimester abortion at that time, prior to and in the early 70's. Saline abortions could only be used during this mid late stage of pregnancy because the uterus is not big enough, or high enough in the abdomen yet to insert the needle and saline solution until 16 weeks gestation. A 6" long needle is placed through the abdominal wall into the woman's uterus. Amniotic fluid from around the fetus is withdrawn and replaced with a strong, caustic saline (salt) solution. This solution is poisonous to the fetus. It changes the ph of its environment so that basic metabolic functions of the fetus fail. It also burns the fetus's skin and its lungs, as the baby inhales and swallows the caustic amniotic fluid. I was assigned to care for 2 young women who had received the saline injection into their uteri the day before. My job was to comfort the women, who were teenagers themselves, and to assist the docs and them in the delivery of their hopefully dead babies. I was not present with the physician for the needle insertion. The fetus usually dies within an hour of the injected saline. It takes approximately 24 to 48 hours after the saline injection for labor to commence. The women are told that when labor starts it will feel like menstrual cramps, maybe stronger. The girls were dressed in hospital gowns and just sat around in their hospital beds, waiting. The girls were free to walk around. Sometimes they would talk to one another, but mostly the woman just kept to themselves. With a saline abortion, labor progresses as usual. It starts out slow then intensifies through the standard phases of labor as the mother's body senses the death of the fetus and works to expel it. She will deliver the tiny dead fetus by the usual vaginal method. The woman is fully awake. She receives no or an epidural anesthesia. The fetus is very small, maybe one pound at the 4th or 5th month of gestation. The mother sits in a semi reclining position on a delivery table. She will see and sometimes watch as the fetus is expelled, just as if she were to deliver a live baby. My job was not only to assist her and comfort her, but also along with an OB resident, most importantly collect, bag and label the POC for delivery to the pathology lab. The "baby" as I choose to call it, is delivered whole, in one piece. I'll always remember the sight of a baby delivered this way. The baby's skin was reddened, like it had a bad sunburn. They were pinker than pink. The term "Candy Apple Babies" was given to these aborted children as their skin is bright red and shiny from the first and second degree skin burns they endured. The fetus likewise gulps the poisoned caustic amniotic fluid and the fluid burns the inside of the baby's mouth and throat as well. The lungs are also scorched as the baby inhales its own tainted amniotic fluid. It suffers (my opinion).

The dead fetus was barely the size of my petite hand. I doubt it even weighed a pound. Its eyes were partially open. It was male. The amniotic sac was withered but clear and he looked to be perfect in form, complete with all of his fingers and toes. I waited with the OB resident until the woman delivered the placenta. It didn't take long, maybe 5 minutes. In my opinion, it was horrible, but it was legal. What made it all the more frightening was that the young teenage girl was terrified. This was her first pregnancy. She trembled with fear with each contraction. She gasped for breath with each cramp, holding it and bearing down as she tried to control the pains of childbirth. I could hardly calm her. The saddest part also, was that she was alone. She had no support, no one to hold her hand. No husband, no boyfriend, no mother. She was a child herself. What should have been a joyous occasion turned into a nightmare for this young girl. As her extremely premature dead baby was delivered, she gazed down to the lifeless scorched mass. Two people were physically and emotionally tortured that day. One for the rest of her life, and the other was already dead. I do not remember the girl's name. She cried crocodile tears, like babies cry. The OB doc just glanced over to me. The teenager looked at me for reassurance. Was it over? I felt as desperate as she was because I didn't know what the hell to do either. I did not ask her about the circumstances of her pregnancy, but I knew this event would forever dominate her existence.

Saline abortions are not performed today, as in years past it was discovered that a high maternal death rate was associated with this method. This method of abortion was introduced by a Romanian abortionist, Abruel, in 1939, and was practiced by the Japanese post WWII. The Japanese quickly discovered that it was an unsafe practice. Its results were disastrous. As many as sixty maternal deaths were reported over a two year span. The Japanese condemned the saline or "instillation" abortion method, as they noted that the caustic saline solution would be rapidly absorbed by the maternal circulation and that this saline solution was just as toxic to the mother as it was to the fetus. But American physicians did not obtain the Japanese results until years later. Information was not given or received as openly and freely as it is in today's rapid internet line of communication. The instillation or saline method of abortion is not usually practiced today in the United States today.

Next came the D & E or formally known as a "Dilation and Evacuation of the POC". This is the technical name for dilating the cervix and then evacuating the contents of the uterus by means of suction. This was the routine abortion procedure preformed in the operating room. This procedure utilizes a suction machine engineered for this specific medical procedure. The machine is square and is about 3 feet high. This method was the norm for abortions during the first and sometimes the very early second trimester of pregnancy. The woman is placed in the lithotomy position, her legs spread and elevated as if she were to actually give birth if she were to carry the fetus to term. All of the women were given general anesthesia. They needed to be completely knocked out, not only for alleviation of any pain, but also so that the woman could not hear the terrifying roaring noise of the abortion suction machine. To me the abortion suction machine sounded like a 737 barreling down a runway that was 20 feet away. The suction pressure of the abortion machine is 20 times greater than an ordinary vacuum cleaner. After the cervix is dilated repeatedly with increasing sizes of stainless steel dilators, the doctor uses an approximately 1 inch in diameter, plastic cannula with a large hole near its top to suck the fetus from its placement on the inside of the uterine wall. It's like plucking a cherry from the stem of a tree. It looks painful. The doctor will move the suction cannula back and forth within the uterus to make sure its opening reaches every spot on the inside wall of the uterus. The contents of the uterus are instantly sucked through the tubing and deposited into a fabric pouch like container atop the suction machine. We as nurses do not usually see the POC as the fabric sac is not transparent. But sometimes the POC will be seen at the end of the procedure if the suction cannula missed an area where the embryo was attached to the uterine wall, as the doctor will do a curettage after the suction procedure. The surgeon uses a curette for the curettage.

A curette is a surgical instrument with a looped blade on the end that is used to scrape the inside of the uterine wall; hence the C part of the term D & C. The "C" stands for curettage. On occasion, the suction cannula will miss a small embryo or fetus and it will be left attached to the uterine wall, only to be scraped out in the curettage phase of the abortion. It was during this stage of the procedure that I saw the real thing, the beginning of life. Believe me, it was no blob of tissue or mucus. What I saw was a tiny being. In a D & C, the scrapings are deposited by the physician into a sterile gauze, which is then gathered up by the nurse and placed into a specimen jar to be sent to the pathology lab. On several occasions, an embryo would be missed by the suction machine and it would be apparent in the scrapings on the gauze from the curettage.

On this one particular day I found a most unusual specimen of POC. By developmental standard charts, I calculated this one particular embryo to be about 9 weeks gestation. It was a perfect textbook picture. It was as big as a small lima bean, around ½ to ¾ inches in length, but its features were exactly as I learned and had imagined for this stage of development. Its eyes were jet black dots. It had tiny stubby arms and legs that still looked like buds. Its fingers on its hands were more distinct than its toes on its feet, as its toes were still webbed and appeared fan shaped like a frogs. Its head was one half its entire body mass, and its spine was curled resembling the letter C. I could discern the embryo's ears on each side of its head. They looked like micro pimples, but they were there. Its skin was colored pink, the shade of a cooked shrimp. I held the tiny embryo in my hands and then between my finger tips. It was smooth, hairless and warm. It was dense. It had mass. It had weight. It was formed. It was perfect and pure! It was here in my hands and it was real. It wasn't a picture that I had to memorize for my anatomy and physiology classes. Despite all the legislative controversy, ethical deliberations and scientific testing as to when life really begins, I was convinced at that exact moment that this little miniscule thing was a tiny human being. There was no question that this tiny entity was life. It was unique and anatomically exact down to the milligram. It was life because if it weren't, it wouldn't have had to have been removed. Its life cycle was deliberately interrupted. It had a presence that could not be denied. It was life because someone made the choice to end it! Someone decided that it must not be allowed to grow and develop into a fuller life form. It was defenseless. How come this embryo or fetus didn't have a choice? I know why; because it couldn't scream loud enough! The squeaky wheel always gets the oil.

I continued to finish scrapping and picking the tissues off of the sponge that contained this patient's products of conception, when I felt another mass in the sanguineous blob of tissue. I was alone now in the OR room. On a hunch, I brushed the bloody mucus from another small bean shaped density. I was shocked. It was another embryo, exactly like the one I just placed into the first specimen container. "Twins!" I thought to myself. My eyes were welled up with tears, but only for the moment as I had to compose myself. After all, I was at work. Maybe sadness is a better term for my feelings. Whatever the names of the emotion I was experiencing, it did not make me feel proud or good about of myself. Even though I did not perform the abortion myself, I assisted. The doctor and the patient had already left the operating room and the patient was probably already in the recovery room. I often wondered if the gynecologist who preformed her abortion ever told her that she was carrying twins. He would certainly get the pathologist's report within the week and he would have to tell her. Both doctor and patient may have already known, as sometimes elevated HCG levels, the hormone detected in the blood stream that confirms pregnancy may have been extra elevated as seen in twinning. Maybe the patient had an ultrasound and maybe she already knew. Since the chart had already left my possession, I was not privy to that information anymore. Were they identical or fraternal? Were they little boys or little girls? Or were they one of each? I could not tell. The sex of an embryo is determined at approximately 6 weeks gestation, but I wasn't looking for any sexual traits, so I don't know. Maybe if I thought to look closely enough I might have been able to detect the sex, but I didn't.

Abortion's Correlation with Breast Cancer

Are we really practicing medicine when we do abortions? Are we thinking of the women, the unborn, or are we thinking about our pockets? The Hippocratic oath comes to mind. This oath is what the father of medicine Hippocrates claimed to rule his practice and what current physicians may also state as their foundation for practicing medicine.

The Hipprocratic oath states: I will follow that system of regime which, according to my ability and judgment, I consider for the benefit of my patients, and abstain from whatever is deleterious and mischievous. I will give no deadly medicine to anyone if asked, nor suggest any such counsel; and in like manner *I will not give to any woman a pessary to produce abortion.*

Obviously, not all of the elements of this oath apply today primarily because abortion is legal in various parts of the world, now in the 21st century. I am not bashing any profession that participates in preforming abortions; however, ominously there are several draw backs regarding women's health care that modern medicine did not anticipate. According to a specific research study, 2nd and 1st trimester abortion is responsible for a > **100%** increased risk of developing breast cancer when induced. Who knew!? Many of these scientific articles were published in the early years post 1973 when the legalization of abortion in the US blossomed, claiming a definite correlations between abortion and breast cancer risk.

In 1981, twelve years after the passage of Roe vs. Wade, a study was done on American women and published in the British Journal of Cancer that reported "abortion appears to cause a substantial increase risk of 140% increased risk of subsequent breast cancer" (Pike MC et al., British Journal of Cancer (1981;43:72-6).

There are oodles of scientific studies demonstrating significant correlation of induced abortion and subsequent breast cancer; however, conversely there are many research articles that report the opposite, which demonstrate that there is no statistically significant increase in BC post induced abortion. It's rather interesting reading. The latter studies claiming no significant association or increased BC risk, claimed that those early research studies from the 1950s and for awhile afterwards linking BC to induced abortion were prone to flawed research study designs. Recent study reviews indicate and found that these early research models were based on "recall bias". Recall bias can alter significance and true measurable results. Recall bias is when a study participant will vividly recall their abortion and she might be looking for a link or cause of her breast cancer; conversely a healthy woman with no breast cancer and who also had an abortion -but she was not counted in the study. Google it and you'll be shocked like I was. There are pros and cons to this controversial religious and political topic of abortion. The biological facts regarding breast cancer's implied increased risk associated with induced abortion are really quite simple to understand. All non-pregnant women are born with immature breast cells that do not mature or become "functional" milk producing ducts and cells /glands until a woman becomes pregnant. While these breast cells are in their immature stage they are vulnerable to cancer. When a woman becomes pregnant her breast tissue enlarges and the cells multiply rapidly in preparation for lactation after the baby is born. It is during these first two trimesters of a woman's pregnancy when the breast cells multiply exponentially. This stage of breast tissue maturation is called 'proliferation'. The pregnant woman's breast tissues and cells do not reach maturity and become able to produce milk until the 3 rd trimester of pregnancy at approximately 32 weeks. It is during this 3rd trimester of pregnancy when a woman's breast glands fully mature and become functional producing milk when her breasts become resistant to cancer. If the pregnancy goes to full term and the child is delivered and the child is breast fed, this protection is compounded. It has been documented in the British Medical Journal Lancet that for each 12 months of breast feeding, a woman can reduce her risk of breast cancer by 4.3%, and 7% for each live birth(Beral, V (2002):Lancet:360:180-95). Conversely, when the pregnancy is forcibly terminated in the 1st or 2 trimester of pregnancy the woman is left with an overabundance of cancer vulnerable breast cells that never come to maturity and never develop the resistance to cancer. This is how elective abortion **supposedly** hurts women's health because it sets up the fertile ground for future breast cancer development. Over the years, many studies using less biased research models were used and the American Cancer Society's most recent claims very clearly state that **induced abortion does not impact breast health or BC development** http://www.cancer.org/docroot/cri/content/cri_2_6x_can_having_an_abortion_cause_or_contribute_to_breast_cancer.asp. Also, the National Cancer Institute concluded, after prospective research studies that there is no link to having an abortion and subsequent BC development (National Cancer Institute. Abortion, Miscarriage, and Breast Cancer Risk. Accessed at www.cancer.gov/cancertopics/factsheet/Risk/abortion-miscarriage on September 2, 2011). Women need to be given accurate and correct information regarding abortion issues so that she can make a truly informed "CHOICE". Hey, I'm PRO-CHOICE, but let me make an 'informed choice' and not a manipulated mistake. Ask questions and demand answers.

I occasionally think to myself of that woman with the aborted twins and if she could have been one of those 31 % of women who regretted having aborted her child. Would she be depressed as they say 65% of those who abort are? Would she try to commit suicide? Would she be followed up for the subsequent development of breast cancer as related to her abortion? These potential psychological and health consequences of abortion need to be communicated to women seeking abortion. A doctor who performs abortions for a living may or may not be financially focused enough to offer alternatives. Abortion might be a quick fix to immediate concerns, but lifelong future psychological and physical health may be compromised. I am not professing one side or the other, but the information regarding abortion's consequences should be made clear and equal from both sides of the fence.

The Roe vs. Wade decision offered an alternative, but at a significant price for many women. Clear pictures of potential psychological & physical consequences need to revealed to the woman and her immediate significant others. Parents, boyfriends, husbands, and lovers need accurate information regarding this issue. Most importantly, an informed choice needs to be made regarding abortion, not an emotional one. I believe that at the very least, abortion counseling needs to be prescribed to those choosing to abort, and especially to teenagers and to those women with little family or significant other support. Planned Parenthood is a good source of information. Illegitimate pregnancy does not carry the stigma as it did in generations before. In the 1920's children who were born out of wedlock had "ILLEGITIMATE" stamped in large red letters across their birth certificates, so anytime you needed to show your birth certificate to anyone you were automatically judged, announcing your heritage to schools, employers, the armed services, and to the rest of the planet. Really, in today's world that is none of anyone's business and I'm glad that practice was eliminated. Conversely, most women who undergo abortion are OK with it. It all depends on the make up of the woman. Many factors will affect a woman's response post abortion, and there is no magic formula to predict who will react in one way or another. Some can handle it better than others, and that's good. After all, abortion is legal here in the US, and in my opinion it's better to be legal and be done under clean and sterile conditions rather than in a back alley. I know of women who have had several abortions, 2, 3, and 4 abortions and they seem to be fine about it.

Speaking of multiple abortions, now there's another topic. I once knew of a coworker, who during our work day told me that she had "another" abortion over the past weekend. I was kind of shocked that she would reveal such personal information to me, as she was just an acquaintance and not a close friend. So I took that moment as an invitation to get her to talk more about her experience and maybe she was secretly wanting to share her feelings about it. She told me that it was her third abortion and the father was the same man, her boyfriend of 5 years. But most puzzling to me was the fact that she was engaged to marry the man. She even flaunted a huge hunk of rock, a 2 karat solitaire on her left ring finger. I asked her, "Why don't you use birth control or why don't you just have the kid?" Repeated abortions on one's uterus are not too smart as each time you have one there's more scarring and that could potentially cause problems in the future. She replied to me as she simultaneously clicked and snapped the chewing gum, "We're not ready yet." I thought to myself, "Ready for what? Is this chick dense? " I almost said to her, but I didn't, "Why don't you take the frigging pill? What's the matter with you?" I didn't understand her reasoning and I don't think I wanted to. I rationalized that it was her choice and her business and not for me to judge. But I do not condone having multiple abortions as a means of birth control like this woman. By having multiple abortions as a means of birth control, you are setting yourself up for risk factors that can be deadly, like infections, bleeding, blood clots, and future fertility problems. I think I've just about seen it all. Most importantly, we need to not judge our sisters, mothers, daughters, aunts, nieces and friends. Just inform them! Never pressure any woman, whether it be your girlfriend, your lover, your wife and especially your daughter into aborting. Having an abortion should be the woman's choice, and no one else's. We need to educate ourselves about abortion-completely, share it with our friends, daughters, sisters, and mothers so we can empower women to make correct and informed choices.

Many schools will not teach about abortion. Therefore I believe that it is paramount that all mothers inform your daughters regarding issues on sex, pregnancy, birth control, and abortion and its consequences first hand from you. If you don't do it, she'll learn the hard way, like on the streets or from her high school girlfriends and that information will almost always be incorrect. And if you feel you do not know enough to teach her, take her to your own gynecologist, nurse practitioner, or health care provider. The Planned Parent Federation of America.org is another institution that provides care to teens and women and can provide a wealth of information. PPFA is listed in your local phone book. WebMD is a good source for information, or Google it!

CHAPTER 11

A PREVENTABLE DEATH

Leo was a nursing assistant in the Unit. It was here that I landed my first job after graduation in 1976. He was a real jokester. He had a wise crack for everything and everyone. He was about 40 years old, tall and lanky and he had this swirl of thick curly red hair atop his head. And entwined into that mane of his was always a filter less Chesterfield cigarette that sat cradled just above his right ear. Leo also had a persistent deep phlegm packed cough. He was a busy worker. There was always some patient he had to assist to turn, pull up, sit in a chair, get back into bed, or transport to wherever the patient needed to be. After every task he would reward himself with a mini break, which consisted of a cup of black coffee and a Chesterfield cigarette. It was 1976. He could smoke one pack of cigarettes during an eight hour shift, and God only knew how much more he smoked when he wasn't working. There were always circles of smoke ensconcing his head. I noticed that one day Leo's voice sounded hoarse, hoarser than usual, like he had laryngitis. I asked him if he had a cold. He said he did not. He continued that he must have caught some "BUG" and his only complaint was this nasty hoarseness in his voice, and an ache in his shoulder running down his right arm. Since his job entailed physically lifting heavy patients, it was plausible that the ache was strictly musculoskeletal. "It's probably nothing", he reassured me. But he didn't have a cold, or a runny or stuffy nose, or any sneezing. His cough was part of his persona. There was no change in that as it was always there. I only saw him for the first six months of my tenure in the SICU; then he disappeared, just vanished like a puff of smoke. In retrospect that was a bad choice of words. I never saw him again. I just figured that he got another job somewhere else. But he didn't. He died. He died of lung cancer. I over heard my colleagues, my fellow nurses and the doctors talking about him. One of the surgical residents told me that Leo was experiencing "hemoptysis" or the coughing up of blood. I never knew he was sick as he didn't look sick to me. He just had that thick cough, and that recent episode of laryngitis. But I remembered something else about Leo and I wondered if anyone else heard this as well. I remembered that frequently I could hear an audible wheeze. At times his wheeze was so loud you didn't need a stethoscope held against his chest to hear it. I could hear the rattling in his chest while he was breathing if I was sitting only 2 to 3 feet away from him. Come to think of it, Leo had suspicious symptoms. His persistent cough was troubling. He had the cough for longer than a couple of months. A persistent cough can be suspicious as an indicator for lung cancer, especially in a long time smoker. But not all coughs are related to lung cancer. I do not want to alarm people. As a matter of fact, most coughs are not related to lung cancer at all. There are many other diseases where a cough is present and there is no lung cancer. For example conditions like seasonal allergies, asthma, bronchitis or congestive heart failure are possible causes of a persistent cough, but unfortunately persistent coughing can also be a late stage symptom when it comes to lung cancer.

Surprisingly and frequently 25% of all lung cancers are discovered accidentally. One time in four, lung cancer is found in patients with no symptoms of lung cancer at all. Their lung cancer is inadvertently found on a routine chest x-ray or a CAT scan performed for some other reason. In these cases, the lung tumor may be small enough and very localized and not yet possible to produce any symptoms. These people are lucky. Sometimes the early lung lesion is referred to as a "coin" lesion, because it is usually no larger than a coin. In the early stages of lung cancer, symptoms of the disease are not apparent. It is not until the later stages of a lung cancer's growth that the tumor or tumors grow so large that they obstruct air flow in the lungs, producing coughing, wheezing, or pneumonias. Lung cancer can also produce chest pain if it compresses against other structures and organs, like the esophagus or nearby nerves that supply sensation to the area. Tumor compression against the esophagus can produce difficulty swallowing as well. Dysphagia is the term used to describe difficulty swallowing and this would be a very late stage symptom. I do not know if my friend Leo had dysphagia. This 25% group of early stage lung cancer patients are the luckiest because their lesions can sometimes and very frequently be successfully treated with surgical removal and very possibly cured. I say sometimes because the overall prognosis or chances of recovery from lung cancer is the least favorable of all cancers. That is because lung cancer grows so silently and spreads so rapidly. Our lungs have an excellent blood supply and are full of millions of capillaries (tiny blood vessels) needed for life sustaining oxygen and carbon dioxide exchange. Thanks to the vascular component of our lungs, this blood pipeline gives easy transport for the metastasis of the lung cancer as well. Subsequently, because of the lung's anatomical perfection, the basement level 5 year survival rate for lung cancer patients is only 11% to 15%, compared to a five year survival rate of 63% for colon cancer, 88% for breast cancer, and 99% for prostate cancer (Medicine Net.com, 2005).

That's the trouble with lung cancer; often times you don't know you have it until it's too late. In retrospect, Leo's doctors discovered that Leo with his persistent cough, wheezing, laryngitis, hemoptysis and right arm and shoulder pain was definitely experiencing suspicious symptoms. Leo's symptoms and history told a text book lung cancer story.

Hemoptysis, or the coughing up of blood in your sputum is a big "RED FLAG" and should be brought to the attention of your healthcare professional immediately to be evaluated. Fortunately, there is one positive side to lung cancer, and that is to know that lung cancer is one of those diseases that is completely and almost 100% preventable if you know what to avoid: CIGARETTE SMOKING AND RADON GAS! Lung cancer is 95% preventable if you don't smoke or are not exposed to radon gas.

According to the National Institute on Drug Abuse (2006), tobacco use is the leading preventable cause of death in the United States. But you already knew that. In 2005 lung cancer accounted for most of the cancer deaths in both men and women worldwide. Lung Cancer is the #1 cancer killer. Subsequently, lung cancer has surpassed breast cancer as the #1 cause of cancer deaths in women. Women need to come to terms with the reality that lung cancer is not a "Man's Disease". According to the National Lung Cancer Partnership (2006), lung cancer kills more women than breast, uterine and ovarian cancers combined. According to the NLCP in 2006, lung cancer affects 80,000 American women annually and over 70,000 of these prove to be fatal. Also, 30,000 more women die annually from lung cancer than from breast cancer (NLCP, 2006). Lung cancer is responsible for 30% of all cancer deaths (The Beverly Fund, 2009). The only good news about lung cancer is that in 2009 the ACS recorded that the incidence of lung cancer has declined by 1%. The ACS determined that the decline in cancer deaths and incidence is due to increased risk reduction by quitting smoking and never starting smoking.

Fewer Americans are smoking. It is approximated that 50 million Americans or 19.8% of the US population presently smoke cigarettes. That's almost 1 in 5 people smoke. As of 2007 for the first time since the mid 1960s when the incidence of smoking was at a whapping 42.4%, now in 2009 the rate of smoking fell below 20% (ACS, 2009). Unfortunately the death rates of lung cancer patients are increasing, primarily because the population is increasing. The death rate is a lagging indicator and might be reflected in the future as the population increases and lung cancers can develop decades after a person quits smoking. We shall see. The important factor is that smoking incidence is decreasing and ultimately the death rate of lung cancer due to decreased smoking will subsequently follow.

Before 1900 lung cancer was unheard of! But its rise has increased a hundred fold since the 1930's as smoking tobacco became popular and stylish in the first half of the 20th century. Also, before the 1930's the ill effects of smoking like lung cancer were not definitively associated with smoking. The connection was not made until mid way through the twentieth century. As early as the 1930's, Nazi Germany scientists associated cigarette smoking with the incidence of lung cancer, but because of its political affiliations the information was not accepted by other nations. The history of tobacco use and smoking cigarettes goes back to the first century. Today's tobacco plants began growing in the Americas as early as 6000 BC. The Aztec Indians from South America were pictured in archeological drawings smoking rolled leaves of tobacco and using pipes. Sects of Mayan Indians from Mexico migrated and settled in the Mississippi Valley and cultivated and used tobacco in its many forms. The Mayans introduced and shared their tobacco customs with their neighboring Native North American tribes. Interestingly, the Mayan term for smoking is "sik' ar" (cigar?). In 1492 when Christopher Columbus landed on the Caribbean island of San Salvador he was greeted by native Arawaks and offered gifts of tobacco leaves. Sailors from Columbus's fleet saw the Arawaks and Taino tribes smoking and took up the habit. Rodrigo de Jerez, a sailor with Columbus is documented and credited with being the first European to take up the habit of smoking. It is stated that he became a confirmed smoker, which to me can also be interpreted as he became addicted to the nicotine. When he returned home to Spain he likewise introduced smoking to his hometown. Later in 1610, in England Sir Francis Bacon revealed insight into tobacco's addictive properties as he writes that, "Tobacco use is increasing and that it is a custom that is hard to quit". Today we know without reservation that nicotine is addictive and that the incidence of lung cancer is directly associated with cigarette smoking. However, it has been known for hundreds of years since the 1700s that smoking was associated with shortened life spans and especially with cancers of the head, neck, and mouth, specifically the jaw and larynx. Doctors and researchers have noted the correlation between smoking and cancer but due to several manipulative reasons by tobacco companies or just denial and maybe some ignorance, the warnings were not received by the masses. In 1941, even the world renown surgeon Dr. Michael Debakey remarked that that there was an increased incidence of lung cancer and smoking. In 1938 Prof. Raymond Pearl from John Hopkin's university department of biology wrote in a paper "Tobacco Smoking and Longevity" documented how smokers die prematurely as compared to non smokers. **87 *Science* (#2253) 216-217 (4 March 1938).** Likewise—**NVSR 49, No. 3, U.S. Centers for Disease Control (6-26-2001) He** confirms his findings and documents how male smokers lost 13.2 years of life and females lost 14.5 years of life as a result of smoking. The CDC confirms that 90% of all lung cancers can be attributed to the smoking of cigarettes. Fortunately we have the pioneering research of the world's most eminent scientist of the twentieth century, Sir Richard Doll to thank for his very timely and startling research, which he documented in the early 1950s, that cigarette smoking was and is the major cause of lung cancer. The talk was out there for hundreds of years but his research in 1954 cemented the facts. Sir Richard Doll, an epidemiologist with Oxford University in England, and his colleague Austin Bradford Hill in 1950 performed a study using a simple 5 question questionnaire to interview 649 lung cancer patients. Doll initially hypnotized that the tarring of the streets in industrializing Great Britain early in the twentieth century was the culprit causing the increasing numbers of lung cancer patients. He stated that "the mortality from lung cancer was increasing every year in the first few decades of the last century." http://news.bbc.co.uk/2/hi/health/4092919.stm. Sir Richard Doll continued also that people did not pay any attention to these mortality rates due to lung cancer during the war (WWII), but in the years that followed they became increasingly concerned. Sir Richard stated also that what compelled him to investigate lung cancer was the fact that lung cancer's mortality rate was increasing at a very rapid rate. At the beginning of the twentieth century lung cancer was a rare disease and between the 1920's and 50's the mortality of lung cancer had increased more than 20 times. "So something was happening" He stated. http://news.bbc.co.uk/2/hi/health/4092919.stm.. Initially tests on animals ruled out the link between cigarette smoking and lung cancer. Sir Richard admitted that he at first suspected that the tarmac used in the paving of the streets was to blame because he stated, "We knew that there were carcinogens in tar." It was at this juncture that Sir

Richard and his associates compiled the research tools and statistical methods needed to demonstrate the common thread. The researchers collected data and interviewed 649 lung cancer patients. Their results were frightening. Of the 649 lung cancer patients interviewed, only 2 were non smokers! The results of his research clearly demonstrated that the most common factor associated with this dreaded disease was that these lung cancer patients overwhelmingly smoked cigarettes, and for a long time. His research was groundbreaking. Sir Richard stated "We asked them everything we could think of." Sir Richard Doll, who himself smoked cigarettes quit smoking two thirds of the way into the study because he was convinced that his own smoking habit would surely kill him if he continued to smoke. He was frightened by his own research. At the time of his presentation to the scientific community, 80% of the adult population of England smoked. His first study was published in 1950 in the "British Medical Journal" and was eventually confirmed in 1954 (Doll, R; Hill, Ab; 1950; Smoking and Carcinoma of the Lung; preliminary report" British Medical Journal, 2; 739-48). http://www.pubmedcentral.nih.gov/articlerender.fcgi?tool=pubmed&pubmedid=14772469.

The rest is history. In January of 1964, the Surgeon General of the United States at that time, Dr. Luther L. Terry, also declared that smoking cigarettes was the leading factor in the development of lung cancer. In 1965 warning labels were printed on one side of each pack of cigarettes manufactured in the United States informing smokers of the link between smoking cigarettes and lung cancer. Additionally, Sir Richard Doll's research revealed that the risk of developing lung cancer increases with the number of cigarettes smoked, the duration of years smoked, and even more interesting, the early age at which one begins smoking. At the same time in 1950, other researchers demonstrated strong correlations between smoking and lung cancer. One such person is Morton Levin, who in May 27, 1950 in JAMA, published the first major study linking cigarette smoking to lung cancer and in the same issue of JAMA another study entitled "Tobacco Smoking as a Possible Etiologic Factor in Bronchiogenic Carcinoma: a Study of 684 Proved cases", by Wydner and Graham in the United States, found that 96.5 % of lung cancer patients interviewed were moderate to heavy chain smokers. Sir Richard Doll's research hauntingly revealed that people who started smoking as teenagers and who continued to smoke into adulthood had the highest incidence of lung cancer. Sir Richard Doll died in July of 2005 at the ripe old age of 92, and NOT OF LUNG CANCER! Today, physicians and researchers alike refer to this time risk in terms of "pack-years" of smoking history. More explicitly, it is the number of packs smoked per day multiplied by the number of years smoked. For example, if a person smokes 3 packs of cigarettes a day for 10 years, 3 X 10 = a 30 pack year history of smoking. The incidence of lung cancer rises even with only a 10 pack year history. This means that by just smoking 1 pack of cigarettes a day for only 10 years is enough to give someone lung cancer. But for those individuals who smoke two or more packs of cigarettes a day, like a 30 pack year history smoker, 1 in 7 of those people will die of lung cancer. A 30 pack year history and above smoker has the greatest risk of developing lung cancer. I can remember reading patients' charts while I was the circulating nurse in lung cancer

OR cases, sitting on a chair reading and being amazed at how much some people smoked. Many of these lung cancer patients had 60, 70, and 80 pack year smoking histories. WOW, that's a lot of cigarettes! If those people only knew at that time of their lives when they started smoking that the habit was going to chop their lives short, then maybe they would have opted to never start. On average, smoking cigarettes cuts 10 years off of your life span. But the good news is that if one quits smoking, each year the risk of developing lung cancer decreases significantly. It is during this non smoking period that our lungs will begin to heal and return to their normal state. Immediately, immediately, immediately normal lung tissue begins to replace damaged and inflamed lung tissue and it is estimated that **after 15 years of quitting smoking, the risk of developing lung cancer reverses and equals that of a non, never smoker, or a "0 pack year" smoking history"!** It is very reassuring to know that it is never too late.

As we all know, misery loves company because lung cancer is not the only evil consequence of smoking tobacco. Cancer of everywhere else in the body, like the throat, mouth, esophageal, larynx, stomach, bladder, kidney (nicotine is excreted in the urine) can be associated with smoking cigarettes. Smoking is highly associated with other deadly diseases too; like heart disease, high blood pressure, and gingivitis just to name a few. I've witnessed with my own OR Eyes the many radical surgeries performed due to cancer involving all of these different organs. To me, the most frightening surgical procedure I saw was a "radical glossectomy", which was the removal of the tongue due to cancer. Of course this person smoked cigarettes. Oh wait, I changed my mind. Another time I was involved in a "laryngectomy" or the surgical removal of one's voice box, which was due to smoking as well. That poor person had to have a permanent tracheostomy performed as well. I'll admit, I smoked cigarettes for approximately 3 to 4 years when I was in nursing school, but after seeing the consequences of smoking cigarettes I went "cold turkey" and quit. After working in an operating room and witnessing the nightmarish outcomes of cancer surgeries, I was literally afraid of ever developing any kind of oral or head and neck cancer and having to undergo such radical and disfiguring surgery. After witnessing such face altering procedures I became a hypochondriac! Living in fear is no way to exist. I must admit, that starting smoking cigarettes is the only thing I've ever regretted in my life; but conversely and happily, quitting smoking was the far better and best thing I ever did in my life!

But quitting smoking is not an easy task. This is because nicotine, the drug present in tobacco is a highly addictive substance. The Report on the Scientific Committee on Tobacco and Health in 1988 concluded that nicotine has been shown to have effects on the brain's dopamine system similar to such drugs as heroin and cocaine, and therefore is just as addictive as these two narcotics. The inhalation of nicotine with its instant delivery to the circulatory system (there's that good blood supply to the lungs again) stimulates the dopamine receptors in our brains to release dopamine. Dopamine is associated with pleasurable sensations. But as one continues to smoke, the nicotine will cause lesser satisfaction and so the smoker needs more nicotine to produce more dopamine for more pleasure and satisfaction. Enter addiction. It is a vicious circle. Concurrently, in 1988 the US Surgeon General reported that it is the nicotine in cigarettes that is the addictive component to smoking. In a survey conducted in 2004 by Lader & Meltzer, 70 % of smokers admit the desire to quit smoking, but have little success. Lader, D and Meltzer, H. Smoking related behaviour and attitudes, 2003, ONS, 2004. Anyone who has ever smoked can attest to the fact that it takes several attempts to break the habit. Only about 3 % of smokers are able to quit "cold turkey". Nicotine's addictive snare is demonstrated by the fact that many smokers are reluctant to quit, even after undergoing radical surgery for smoking related cancers. According to Stolerman & Jarvis (1995), about 40 % of patients who have had a laryngectomy (surgical removal of the larynx or voice box,) try smoking soon afterwards, and about 50 % of lung cancer patients resume smoking soon after undergoing lung removal surgery. (Stolerman, IP & Jarvis, MJ., "The scientific case that nicotine is addictive", Psychopharmacology 1995; 117: 2-10). http://www.cdc.gov/tobacco/quit_smoking/you_can_quit/nicotine.htm.

My friend Leo was never a candidate for surgical removal of his lung cancer because the tumor had extended beyond his chest. His tumor or tumors were impinging on other structures within his chest. Only 10-35% of lung cancer patients are eligible for surgical excision of their tumors because of this reason. Leo's tumor had spread to his bronchus, trachea or wind pipe and for obvious reasons theses patients cannot have these structures removed, at least completely. Leo exhibited hoarseness of his voice which was symptom of his lung cancer. He did not have laryngitis but he was experiencing paralysis of his vocal cords due to the cancerous tumors compressing against nerve bundles in his chest that innervated his vocal cords. Recently, in 2006 a famous newscaster named Peter Jennings also fell victim to lung cancer. He also was a previous cigarette smoker. Mr. Jennings also demonstrated the apparent late stage symptom of hoarseness of his voice due to tumor compression on structures affecting his vocal cords. He stated this fact on the his TV broadcast. I watched it. My friend Leo only received palliative or pain relieving and comfort measures for his cancer until he died. He was basically a hospice patient at the time of his diagnosis. He was not a candidate for other medical treatments. But note also that this was in 1976. Chemotherapy and radiation therapies at that time had only moderate success in treating lung cancer, especially if diagnosed in its later stages, which many lung cancers were or are. Cyber knife was not an option 35 years ago. Leo lived for 10 weeks after his diagnosis.

When I would scrub in on a lung cancer case in the OR, it was always sad. The patients were so scared. They were afraid of the lung cancer as well as going under the knife. What I noticed about the lungs imbedded with cancerous tumors was dramatic compared to healthy normal lung tissue. Normal lungs are smooth and have a pale pinkish/pale whitish color, but lungs affected with cancer are just dirty looking. Some lungs with cancerous tumors were jet black with lumps of colorful red and purple tumors. But there's more. When the surgeon would finish excising out the affected lobe, he or she would pass it to me, and I would place it into a shiny sterile stainless steel pan, and if I passed the specimen close enough to my masked face I could smell the stench of wet cigarette tobacco. I guess it was the smell of nicotine. Healthy lungs look clean, and fresh and spongy. If people could see what I've seen with my OR Eyes they would never smoke. The damage to the inside of our bodies caused by nicotine and cigarette smoking is profound.

Unfortunately, one does not have to have a smoking history to develop lung cancer. 15% of lung cancer patients never smoked. There are other risk factors that contribute to the 15% of lung cancer deaths not associated with smoking. Radon gas exposure, & asbestos inhalation otherwise known as mesothelioma, and passive smoking of second hand smoke are guilty culprits as well. Passive smoking refers to the inhalation of tobacco smoke from others who smoke in the same living or working environment as the non smoker. Research has shown that a non smoker who resides with a smoker, has a 24% increased risk for the development of lung cancer, as compared to someone who lives with a non smoker. The CDC calculates there are 3,000 lung cancer deaths a year associated with passive smoking. But there is a more alarming statistic regarding this disease. Radon (Rn) gas exposure is worse!

Exposure to radon gas ranks higher than passive smoking and asbestos exposure as a risk factor for the development of lung cancer. The World Health Organization (WHO) in 2010 stated that exposure to radon gas is the second leading cause of lung cancer, not passive smoking in non -smokers, as is popularly thought. Exposure to radon gas is the #1 cause of lung cancer in people who do not smoke. While smoking cigarettes is responsible for 160,000 lung cancer deaths yearly in the US, the development of lung cancer due to radon exposure comes in at a not too shabby 2nd place with 21,000 yearly deaths. Lung cancer deaths due to radon exposure account for 12% of lung cancer deaths. Of these 21,000 radon deaths, 2,900 of these lung cancer patients never smoked.

Exposure to radon gas can occur anywhere. It can take place in the home or in the work place.

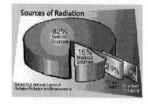

Radon gas is a radioactive gas that is odorless and colorless, and tasteless. Radon (Rn) is chemically inert and essentially non-reactive with other elements. It is one of those noble gasses we learned about in chemistry class. Radon's atomic weight is 84 and can be found in the vertical column furthest to the right in the periodic table. Radon gas is found in soil and ground water in every state in the United States, as well as worldwide. Radon is a naturally occurring gas caused by the decay of uranium in the soil and rock formations. It mixes readily with the air and ground water, especially cold water. Radon gas is a form of radiation and is a potent carcinogen, especially in high concentrations of amounts of 4p/Ci L or higher. When released into the air, radon dissipates rapidly, and instantly into non harmful amounts of radiation. Radon is a naturally occurring element and is evident as normal background radiation. This background radiation accounts for 82% of our radon exposure and is harmless to humans. It measures in very small amounts in the atmosphere.

Radon becomes harmful to people when it seeps into our homes and concentrates indoors where we inhale it into our lungs. Radon gas silently and dangerously enters into homes easily through cracks in our homes' foundations and through ground water via its pipes, if the home uses well water. Radon levels are higher in the lowest levels of a house, like the basement. The closer to the source (in the ground/soil) the bigger the dose you receive. Sometimes we ingest it, especially if one drinks well water that sits atop soils or rocks which emit the radon gas into it as the uranium decays. This route of absorption of radon, via the stomach is responsible for substantial numbers of stomach and esophageal cancers. Like wise, if we routinely shower with well water that is contaminated with radon, it will pose increased risk in the development of lung cancer, as the radio active gas which was dissolved in the water is released into your immediate vicinity or shower upon exposure to the air. January is "Radon Awareness Month" because it is during this cold month that we seal up our homes to prevent the escape of heat, when radon levels are at their peak levels. Radon gas in higher concentration over 4p/Ci L is cause for concern. In 2005, Dr. Richard H. Carmona, the Surgeon General of the United States issued a national health advisory on Radon. Newer homes are routinely inspected for harmful radon levels, but in older homes it is the home owner's responsibility to check for increased radon levels. Home radon detection kits are easy to use and they can be purchased at your local hardware store for under $35.00. Home Depot and Lowes home improvement centers, neighborhood hardware stores carry these kits.

When released into the air, radon dissipates into negligible amounts.. Radon easily diffuses through rock and soil. It is readily soluble in cold water. There are specific rocks and soils that naturally contain high levels of uranium and natural deposits of radon. These areas are where significant deposits of granite, shale, pitchblende, and phosphate are located. Geographic locations where significant recent glacial activity has been documented, in the last 10,000 years are ground zeros for uranium deposits and radon emissions. Below is a current EPA map of the United States which depicts regions of varying levels of radon emissions.

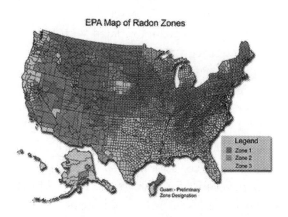

The Midwest section of the United States has the most intense environmental radon concentration due to these glacial deposits. If one recalls their grade school geography classes, the Great Lakes were carved out of the soil and rock by these glaciers. The Appalachian mountain range which runs through the states of Pennsylvania and New York, Maryland, Virginia and Tennessee have high levels of radon emissions as well. The Eastern Seaboard coastal regions of the US, Florida and the entire Gulf of Mexico coastal areas have lower levels of radon emissions.

People who are ate risk for excessive radon exposure are found everywhere. Specifically, miners who work in uranium mines located in the western US states and Canada are at increased risk. In the United States, the state of Iowa has the highest levels of ground radon emissions, but somewhere in every state in the US has dwellings where measured radon levels exceed the acceptable limit of 4 p Ci/L. The Environmental Protection Agency (EPA) estimates that 6% of American homes (approximately 6 million homes) have indoor radon levels above the 4 p Ci/L limit. Since radon gas is as ubiquitous as it is undetectable, the only way to detect it is to have your home tested for it. You have to do it yourself.

This incidence of lung cancer associated with radon gas was first discovered in the 16th century. It was not known as lung cancer at that point in time, but as the "wasting disease" of many miners, as it was recorded by Paracelsus and Aricola. In 1879 this "wasting disease" was described as "lung cancer" by Herting and Hesse who investigated these miners and their sickness. But the element gas "radon "was not discovered until 20 years later by Rutheford. Eventually the connection was made between the miners, radon gas exposure and the incidence of lung cancer. Miners have an increased risk of developing lung cancer because of the higher concentrations of radon gas inhaled and present in unventilated confined mines.

Also, exposure time as dictated by the long work day, often 8 hours or more increases the length of time exposed to the deadly gas. Today, miners don elaborate head gear equipped with filtering air systems to eliminate this risk of radon inhalation. Tragically, smoking cigarettes poses an increased risk for the development of lung cancer in miners as tobacco smoke exponentially and synergistically increases the risk of lung cancer occurrence.

Interestingly, pockets of non smokers who developed lung cancer were noted to be living in geographic locations with higher than usual radon emissions into their homes. Home radon levels are usually higher in colder climates (winter) than in the warm south (spring and summer months) as in the colder climates homes are closed up to keep warm air inside and likewise have less ventilation to the outside air. Radon gas dissipates into harmless levels immediately upon its release into the atmosphere. Besides miners, other occupational workers/individuals who are at risk for developing lung cancer due to inhalation of radon gas are:

1. Mine workers of uranium, hard rock, & vanadium

2. workers remediating radioactive contaminated sights

3. workers at underground nuclear waste sights

4. radon mitigating contractors and testers

5. employees of natural caves

6. phosphate fertilizer plant workers

7. oil refinery workers

8. underground utility workers

9. subway tunnel workers

10. construction excavators

11. power plant workers

12. employees of radon health mines

13. employees of radon balneotherapy spas

14. water plant operators

15. fish hatchery attendants

16. employees who come in contact with naturally occurring radioactive substances

17. people who have incidental exposure from any occupation (WHO,2005).

The best information I can give to any one regarding radon gas and its potential negative impact on our health is to have your home checked for excessive radon concentrations. Radon detection is cheap and easy, and the elimination of radon from your home can be just as cheap and easy. Sealing up cracks in your basement's and your home's foundation might be the most expensive remediation. Adequate ventilation may also be needed to reduce levels of harmful radon gas. In today's climate of energy conservation and tightly sealed up homes to prevent the escape of expensive heating fuels, it is also prudent to know that there are companies who specialize in radon remediation. You can call your local utility company and ask who to call and where to go to seek these services. Lung cancer due to exposure to radon gas can be 100% preventable if we only become knowledgeable of its existence, its prevalence and take measures to avoid and eliminate it.

Exposure to second hand smoke or "passive smoking" is the third leading cause of lung cancer. The WHO (2005) states that lung cancer caused by passive smoking is responsible for approximately 3,000 deaths yearly in the US. One thousand of these lung cancer deaths were of people who never smoked, and the remaining 2,000 lung cancer deaths were to people who smoked previously, but were not smoking at the time of their deaths.

Who Should Be Evaluated for Lung Cancer?

Any person, especially a cigarette smoker experiencing any of the follow symptoms should consult your health care professional.

1. A new persistent cough or worsening of an existing cough
2. Blood in your sputum
3. Persistent bronchitis or repeated respitory infections, pneumonias
4. Chest pain
5. Unexplained weight loss and or fatigue
6. Breathing difficulties such as shortness of breath
7. Difficulty swallowing
8. Wheezing
9. Unexplained hoarseness of voice

But preventing lung cancer is the easier route to travel to avoid this disease. That old saying "An ounce of prevention is worth a pound of cure" is key when it comes to lung cancer. **If you don't smoke, don't start!** Cigarette smoking is a form of nicotine addiction. Going "Cold Turkey" has a low success rate for quitting, so be proactive and admit it and get assistance from a health care professional or support from family members. **Lung cancer is 95% preventable**!!!!! Stopping smoking if you are smoking presently is of paramount importance in the prevention of lung cancer. The damage to your lungs is reversible and your lung cancer risk can revert to a never smoker status! There are many products available that can be purchased to aid in the process of quitting. Likewise, limit your expose to second hand smoke.

Have your home tested for radon emissions. Eliminating radon from your home can be accomplished quickly, most times easily and most times very economically.

CHAPTER 12

PREVENTION BY DIET

Living healthy by eating a healthy diet is probably the cornerstone to preventing all chronic and serious diseases like cancer. Eating fresh fruits and vegetables have always played an important role in preventing all types of cancer, but recent research published in the Lancet, has demonstrated that specifically consuming cruciferous vegetables has decreased the risk of developing lung cancer in smokers. Cruciferous vegetables contain the compound substance *isothiocyanate*. Isothiocyanates have demonstrated to have chemotherapeutic effects against all kinds of cancers, but significantly against lung cancer. Isothiocyanates have sulfur containing photochemicals which have strong chemopreventitive properties against lung cancer. These sulfur compounds neutralize carcinogens rendering them harmless. However there is a genetic component to this miraculous effect. The human genes GSTM1 and GS1T1 normally bind with isothiocyanates and usher them out of our bodies. It is this portion of the human population that has the inactive forms of these genes who benefit the most from the anti-cancer effect of cabbage and who have increased levels of isothiocyanates and a lesser cancer risk by 35%. So the answer is that unless you know if you have the inactive form of these genes, it is recommended to increase your consumption of the cruciferous family of vegetables regardless. The cruciferous family of vegetables include: cabbage, broccoli, cauliflower, kale, turnips, collards, Brussels sprouts, radish, and watercress. So, Opt for the coleslaw (cabbage) instead of the French fries at your next fast food stop.

Omega 3 Fatty acids which are found in abundance in cold water fish like, salmon, herring, halibut, and sardines are essential components of a cancer fighting and preventing diet. Fry it, broil it, or bake it. Just eat it: 2 sevings a week is recommended. **Serve sushi as an appetizer instead** of dips (mayo-high fat) and chips (no nutritive value!)

Drink at least eight 8 oz. glasses of ionized water daily. Water keeps everything moving and flushes waste material from our bodies via the kidneys. Ionized water alkalinizes your body and cancer cannot live in an alkaline environment (ph over 7.5). Cancer thrives in an acidic environment (ph under7.5). Eating junk foods, processed foods, red meat, and sugar produce acid environments in our bodies and thus feed cancers. Fresh fruits and vegetables produce an alkalinizing atmosphere in our bodies and all have antioxidant properties that help fight cancers. *Fruits and vegetables with the most intense colors have the most anti-cancer effects*. For example: Munch on blueberries, blackberries, red and black grapes, strawberries, figs, pumpkin, carrots, and any green veggie.

Tomatoes for example are power houses chock full of anti oxidant cancer fighting substances. The photo nutrient lycopene is a carotenoid and it has been studied in humans abundantly. Lycopene prevents damage to cells and other structures from oxygen, and it protects our DNA molecules or our genetic material as well. Lycopene has also demonstrated protection from heart disease. Lycopene has also demonstrated protection against prostate cancer, breast cancer, intestinal cancers, endometrial cancer, lung cancer, and pancreatic cancer, but especially when consumed with fatty foods such as olive oil, avocadoes, or nuts. This effect is due to the fact that carotenoids, like lycopene are fat soluble and are more readily absorbed into our bodies if eaten along with fats.. Vitamins A (carotenoid),D,E, & K are fat soluble vitamins and are stored in the fat of our bodies.

A funny story related to fat soluble vitamins comes to mind. When I was in nursing school my roommate Sandy developed a weird physical ailment related to her diet. Sandy was always experimenting with different diets in order to lose those last 10 extra pounds. She finally settled on a diet that consisted almost entirely on cantaloupes. Cantaloupes are a sweet fruit and packed with many vitamins and minerals, especially Vitamin A. The carotenoids in Vitamin A give it its orange color, like a carrot. One day Sandy woke up and came storming into my side of the dorm suite and said to me "Kathy, Look at me! I'm jaundiced!" My eyes popped wide open and my jaw dropped. She was right. She looked like she went swimming in a tub full of orange Kool-Aid. She was orange from head to toe. Even the sclera of the eyes was yellow/orange. She was so orange that the palms of her hands were stained bronzed orange as well. She ran over to the ER at MCP to see a doctor. She was sure she had hepatitis. I was afraid for her too. After a 5 hour wait in the ER and undergoing testing she returned back to our dorm. "What did they say it was"? I asked her. "I have HYPERCAROTINOSIS!" she yelled. "What's that?" I asked. "It's from eating too many cantaloupes. I have too much Vitamin A from the excess intake of beta carotenes contained in the cantaloupe from my diet. It gets stored in the fat cells of my body and it turned my skin orange, like the color of a cantaloupe, or a carrot!" It took about a month for her skin to return back to normal. She was lucky because hypercarotenosis due to ingesting too much beta carotenes via diet is a benign condition and there were no long term effects; She just the looked weird for a month! This is my favorite college roommate story. I still laugh out loud today when I think of Sandy and her cantaloupe diet.

Anyway, tomato eaten in any form is acceptable. Cooking does not affect the lycopene content of tomatoes. Raw tomatoes, tomato sauce, stewed tomatoes, even ketchup contains significant amounts of the anti-cancer agent lycopene.

Lycopene is also found in hefty amounts in watermelon, pumpkin, plums, persimmon, pepper, peach, paw paw, mango, guava, grapes, grapefruit, red berry, cloud berry, orange, the leaves of tea, and in the roots of radish, carrots,and cabbage. Lycopene gives these fruits and vegetables their red color. http://www.ivychem.com/extract/lycopene.htm.

All fruits and vegetables contribute to a healthy body and I only used tomatoes as an example of how powerful one fruit can be. The literature is packed with charts on all the benefits given by these important food stuffs so just Google it and see for yourself and choose your favorite ones to incorporate into your personal healthy diet.

- Blueberries are another deeply colored fruit that is a power house when it comes to neutralizing free radicals. Blueberries are packed with antioxidants, of the photo nutrients called anthocyanins. These anthocyanins neutralize free radical damage to the collagen matrix of cells and tissues that can lead to cataracts, glaucoma, peptic ulcers, varicose veins, hemorrhoids, heart disease, and cancer. Researchers at Tufts University analyzed 60 fruits and vegetable for their anti oxidant activity and it was found that blueberries ranked at the top. Tufts University. Researching a Blueberry/Brain Power Connection. Tufts University Health and Nutrition Letter, March 2001, Vol. 19. Number 1 2001

- In another study published in the Archieves of Opthamology, researchers found that by eating just 3 servings of fruits and vegetables a day will lower your risk of developing age related macular degeneration by 36 %. Cho E, Seddon JM, Rosner B, Willett WC, Hankinson SE. Prospective study of intake of fruits, vegetables, vitamins, and carotenoids and risk of age-related maculopathy. *Arch Ophthalmol.* 2004 Jun;122(6):883-92., PMID:

- 15197064

Clearly, these two vividly colored fruits and vegetables pack a huge punch against fighting free radical damage and in preventing all types of illness, including many cancers. Conversely, taking vitamin supplements are expensive and they do not equal the effects of the real fruits and vegetables. Fresh fruits and vegetables contain other nutrients, chemically reactive substances, and minerals that work synergistically with each other to potentate their beneficial effects. The Vitamin and nutrient values for the fruits and vegetables discussed here were referenced at www.healthalternatives2000.com.

Fruits and vegetables are also excellent sources of fiber. Diets high in fiber like whole grains, fruits, vegetables, and legumes promote colon health as they facilitate foods propulsion through the colon thereby preventing constipation. Fiber also help to provide or the feeling of fullness and can help with weight management because it takes longer to chew high fiber foods thereby slowing down the amount of food stuffs consumed. High fiber diets also are also "less energy dense" which means less calories consumed in relation to large amounts of food consumed. Diets high in fiber also promote lowering cholesterol levels because they lower LDL bad cholesterol. Diets rich in fiber also help to reduce blood pressure because of the reduction of LDL cholesterol and decreasing inflammation. Amounts of Fiber recommended for men and women are as follows:

Men;   Over 50 31 gms of fiber
                Under 50 38 gms of fiber

Women;	Over 50 25 gms of fiber
	Under 50 21 gms. Of fiber

www.Mayoclinic.com/health/fiber (2010).

So choose your fruits and vegetable colorfully.

The darkest color vegetable I can think of that most recently has been documented as having the most anti-cancer compounds, anti-oxidants, flavonoids than any known food substance on Earth to date is "CHOCOLATE"! Yes you heard me, that rich creamy yummy stuff that we pour over our desserts and which is infused into hundreds of food stuffs. It really isn't a vegetable, but it is classified as one. Chocolate is extracted from the seeds of the pulpy fruit of the Cacao tree.. Chocolate comes from the seeds inside the cocoa bean plant. Cocoa trees have grown wild in the tropical jungles of the Amazon basin for 10,000 years and were first cultivated by the Olmec Indians as far back as 1,500 years ago. http://www.thenibble.com/reviews/main/chocolate/the-history-of-chocolate.asp. Their neighbors the Aztec and Myans also enjoyed the fruits of the plant. These naïve Americans drank chocolate daily. Chocolate is liquid at room temperature. The Myan word for chocolate is "Xocoatl", pronounced "sho-kwa-til". That sounds pretty close to how we in the 21st century say it. The cacao beans' extract, this chocolate was introduced to the European explores 500 years ago. The rest is history. Chocolate sucks up the free radicals that cause our bodies to age faster, and that cause heart disease, and cancer. Chocolate contains 8 X more of the antioxidants than strawberries. The flavonoid chemicals found in chocolate help to relax the blood vessels thereby helping to lower blood pressure. But the trick to consuming chocolate as a health product is to make sure it is **"DARK CHOCOLATE",** not milk chocolate or white chocolate, which really isn't chocolate at all. It's the cacao bean's dark color that gives chocolate its dark brown black color. Black is Beautiful! Remember the darker and more intense in color your fruits and vegetables are the more nutrient and vitamin packed they are. Dark chocolate also helps to reduce cholesterol. Dark chocolate contains the good fats that help to reduce cholesterol, like oleic acid and stearic acid. Dark chocolate has 65% more cocoa content. http://longevity.about.com/od/lifelongnutrition/p/chocolate.htm. Milk chocolate contains milk which negates or cancels out the positive effects of the cocoa bean rendering it with **"0" ZERO** health benefits. So stick with the dark chocolate.

Studies document eating or drinking 3.5 oz of dark chocolate a day will provide 400 calories, and will enable you to reap the benefits of chocolate. One draw back is that chocolate is high in fat content, but it is good fat, and therefore calorie content is high as well, so always count your calories and exercise to keep that BMI at 25 or a little less.

CHAPTER 13

Oops!

Everyone makes mistakes, but hopefully not in the OR. Some mistakes are minor without any apparent consequences, but some mistakes can be atrocious. In researching this topic I discovered that wrong patient, wrong- site, wrong-side, and wrong -procedure mistakes happen more commonly than what is made known to the public. Every hospital has encountered this scenario and has been sued over some kind of wrong patient, wrong site surgical situation. Slip-ups can occur in all areas of medicine, ranging from reading the wrong X-Rays, mixing up patient records, wrong drug calculations, wrong patient administration of medications, and mixing up biopsy results resulting in incorrectly diagnosing patient diseases, or most tragically, operating on the wrong patient! Amputating a wrong leg, removing or operating on the wrong-side organ (breast, kidney, ovary), inserting a chest tube into the wrong side lung, or irradiating the wrong organ are examples of wrong -site or procedure / surgeries. There are hundreds of documented mistakes that most medical establishments do not want to talk about.

I read about a scenario where two patients had prostate biopsies, and the specimens were mixed up and mislabeled by OR personnel. One patient's prostate biopsy was diagnosed as cancer and the other patient's biopsy was read by the pathologist as a benign condition. Therefore, each gentleman received a wrong diagnosis. The patient who did not have cancer underwent a total radical prostatectomy, a very extensive surgical procedure, and the patient who really had a cancerous prostate gland was discharged and was walking around unknowing of his true medical condition.

According to Health.com, an article stated from a study in the journal "Archives of Surgery", that in a hospital in Colorado over a 6.5 year period, surgeons reported operating on a wrong patient 25 times and operating on a wrong body part 107 times. But these numbers were only the errors that were reported. Also reported was that only 0.5% of medical malpractice suites nationwide involved wrong- site, wrong –side, wrong-procedure, and wrong patient events (WSPE). WSPE's are rare, but they are more common than admitted.

All of these medical mistake scenarios can be attributed to and traced back to some form of **lack of communication or mis-communication.** It happens. I saw it with my own **OR EYES** and it happened on my watch.

I was a nurse manager in an OR on the 3pm to 11 pm shift when this mistake happened. I was not the scrub nurse or the circulating nurse in the OR suite where it happened, and the mistake most likely happened just as I showed up for my shift. The OR case started at the change of shift, when new personnel came on board. It was about 5:00 pm in the afternoon when I got a page from the circulating nurse in the ENT suite. The acronym ENT stands for ear, nose & throat. The ENT suite is where all ENT surgeries were performed. Surgeries like tonsillectomies, larynx procedures, tracheostomies, ear surgeries or surgeries on the tongue and mouth and endoscopic procedures as well were all performed in the ENT suite. The room was equipped with special ENT instruments and supplies. When I returned my page to the circulating nurse in the ENT suite, she answered screaming to me, "GET IN HERE, GET IN HERE!" "OH NO", I thought to myself. I could not imagine what hell I would be walking into. I ran to the ENT suite, swiftly opened the door and witnessed the ENT surgeon throwing OR drapes all over the place, ripping the drapes from the anesthetized OR patient and him screaming, "What the FUCK! What the FUCK! What the FUCK! I asked the circulating nurse, "What happened? What is he screaming about?" The circulating nurse replied, "He operated on the wrong ear. The permit was signed for a Right side stapedectomy, but he did a Left sided stapedectomy." The stapes is one of 3 small bones in the middle ear that helps conduct sound waves. The surgeon discovered the mistake when the surgery was completed and as he was removing the surgical drapes from around the patient's head, that he realized he performed the surgery on the wrong side. After the surgeon calmed down, he finished dressing the patient's ear, and when the patient started to regain consciousness from the general anesthesia, the patient was transported to the recovery room or the **RR**. The mistake was made probably when the patient was received into the OR suite and the circulating nurse, and or the ENT residents, and or the ENT surgeons mistakenly prepped the wrong side ear because they didn't take the time and check the OR permit and compare it to where they were supposed to prep and position the patient's head for the surgical procedure. The patient was already anesthetized. Everyone in that room, especially the OR staff that started the surgery and the people who were responsible for checking the operative permit immediately before the surgery began should have picked up they were prepping the wrong side. The anesthesiologist who also should have checked the permit as well, and who was sitting at the patient's head administering the anesthesia for the 2 hour surgical procedure while monitoring the patient's vital signs should have or could have detected they were operating on the wrong side also. Everyone screwed up that day! In my opinion, it was a team effort! I say this sarcastically, as it was not funny. Just think about it. What if that patient was to undergo a breast mastectomy for breast cancer and she had the wrong breast removed????!!!!!! Or what if the patient was to undergo a below the knee amputation due to the ravages of diabetes and they amputated the wrong leg????!!!!! This kind of mistake is tragic to say the least, no matter what kind of surgery anyone has. Everyone in that OR was freaking out!

That patient returned to the OR the next week and she had her stapedectomy performed on the correct side. What consequences she suffered due to the mistake of operating on the wrong ear, that information I was not privy to and I do not know. If she sued the surgeon, or the residents, or the anesthesiologist, or the hospital or the OR nurses for any damages I do not know that either.

Every surgeon and probably every OR nurse has some recollection of an OR mistake resembling this event. We as health care professionals are acutely aware of medical mistakes as it is an integral portion of any doctors' or nurses' professional training. Some medical mistakes can be life altering. But these kinds of medical mistakes, especially in the OR are **100% completely preventable**. Some methods to prevent these scenarios, and the one I like the most is the "TIME OUT" practice. When OR personnel are getting ready to perform an operation or any procedure, everyone should just stop, step back and verbally confirm to each other exactly what they are going to do:

1. Patient name. **Identify** the patient is the same person wearing the ID bracelet he or she is wearing. Also, while the patient is awake, ask the patient his name and compare it to the ID bracelet he or she is wearing. This makes sure you have the right patient.

2. **Check** the operative permit. Make sure the operative permit is signed by the person in front of you, and ask the patient **exactly** what procedure he or she is having done, **and on which side.**

3. **Confirm** the body part that is being operated on, both verbally and visually. Is the patient having an ovary removed or is the patient having an appendectomy? Both procedures are located in the same proximity on the abdomen.

4. **Label** the area if possible with an indelible marker.

Take the time to be sure.

The American Academy of Orthopedic Surgeons initiated a program entitled **"Sign Your Site",** where the patient and doctors use an indelible marker to "MARK" the correct surgical site to be operated on. At the OR where I worked, all the orthopedics cases /patients came to the OR with Sharpie documented areas instructing the surgeon where to cut. It sounds cute at first, but we were really saving ourselves a lot of headaches regarding the issue of wrong-patient, wrong-side, wrong-site procedure malpractice suits. For example; the total knee replacement patients arrived to the OR with a Sharpie documented Happy Face on the correct knee joint to be replaced and a big giant red X on the knee not to be operated on, as well as text stating; DO NOT CUT HERE! Don't laugh because it works. **Communication is the key** in preventing these types of errors.

In my research regarding this topic of Wrong-patient, wrong-side, wrong- surgical procedure, I found an article published by the National Practitioner Data Bank and documented in the Archives of surgery, 2006; 141: 931-939, and the American Medical Association, Selden, MD(2006), according to its research the causes of these types of errors are as follows:

1. High work load environment

2. Fatigue

3. Multiple team members

4.   Diffusion of authority and lack of accountability

5.   Team communication

6.   Change of personnel

7.   Haste

8.   Incompetence

9.   Inexperience

10. Other.

Any and all of these above reasons for the WSPE I witnessed could be attributed as the cause of the error above, as it occurred at the end of a long day, at the change of shift, and with a boat load of OR professionals who were fatigued and probably just assuming that the other person knew what they were doing, and that they-the other person did the checking, so they didn't have to. **Lack of Team communication** was the most likely and the single biggest factor regarding this event, in my opinion.

Patients be aware of these issues. We are all patients at some time in our lives. All patients have rights that must be upheld. If you feel that a mistake or error was made there are steps you can take.

First, #1. Ask your doctor for an explanation of what and why something happened.

Next, #2 Get a copy of your medical records. You can get these because they are yours. You have a right to see your files and records. Ask questions and demand answers. It's your legal right to do so.

#3, Keep your own records. Document dates, times, names, medicines, tests and procedures performed and their outcomes.

#4 If you are not satisfied by your doc's answers, ask to speak to someone above him/her. The person to ask for is an **Ombudsman,** or a patient advocate at the hospital. If no satisfaction is obtained here, you have a legal right to file a complaint. If your issues are not resolved you can file a complaint at the local and state health departments, or file a complaint to the Joint Commission @ www.jointcommission.org/GeneralPublic/Complaint).

#5 If all else fails, you can consult an attorney.

Conclusions

These are the stories of real OR events, and patients as I knew them. The one lesson that I hope everyone can take with them after reading this book is that all of these OR cases are tragically real and that they are the worst case scenarios that I have encountered, but each and every one of them begs to tell a story on how their diseases could have been prevented, or at least managed successfully if detected early. If only these patients had known, or if someone would have told them what they could have or should have done, their stories would have had more positive outcomes. All of our bad habits, our addictions, our ignorance, our accidents, our denial, our flat out refusals, and or our weaknesses all contributed to the scenarios documented here. Some diseases took us by surprise and caught us all off-guard, like AIDS in the early 80's. How could we have known that AIDS was lurking in the crawl spaces of our lives, right under our noses and that it would rip the complacency and security from our minds only to devastate millions of families and the planet forever. If AIDS would have happened just one century before it did, say in the 1800's, the entire human population as we know it could have possibly been wiped out, as the study of "virology" and viruses didn't even exist yet. Life is a learning process, but it is so much easier to learn from past mistakes or OPMs and learn how to not repeat them.

These "OR Eyes" have seen it all and so I preach to all human beings these health promoting guidelines, the same I preach to my own family, so if you want to avoid a trip to the OR and live a longer and healthier life:

1. Don't' smoke

2. Quit smoking

3. Get your house tested for radon

4. Practice safe sex; avoid risky behaviors; abstinence is an option

5. Get tested for HIV

6. Get your yearly mammogram. Get yearly breast exams. Know your breasts.

7. Don't drink, or text and drive.

8. Sign a donor card.

9. Limit alcohol consumption. Get help if addicted

10. Say NO to drugs. Get help if addicted.

11. Set a BMI of 25 or a little less as your goal. Achieve waist circumference goal of less than 35 inches for women, or less than 45inches for men

12. Lose weight and prevent onset of Type II DM; Modify your diet; Limit white sugar, No processed foods ; Limit high fat content foods.

13. Move your body regularly: walk, swim, pump iron, stretch, jump rope, walk your dog, Hoola –Hoop, or do whatever you can and do for 20 minutes a day.

14. Eat 5 to 7 servings of fruits and vegetables a day. Mix them up. The more deeply colored vegetables and fruit are, the better they are for you. Eat 2 or more servings of cruciferous vegetables like broccoli, cabbage, brussel sprouts, or cauliflower a week.

15. Be aware of abortion issues. Never force any woman to abort.

16. Colonoscopy screening starting at age 50 and every 10 years for early detection of colon polyps/cancers. All colon cancers start as little benign polyps and so colon cancer too is close to 100% preventable.

17. Don't forget to reward yourself with treats like Dark Chocolate !

18. Wear your seatbelt every time you get into a car.

The scenarios portrayed here in "OR Eyes" were probably the most common afflictions affecting hospital surgical patients when I worked there, yet they were sometimes the most unbelievable circumstances that I encountered in my OR and nursing career. Colon cancer is another topic and surgery I participated in frequently, however, the colon cancer surgeries I participated in were not unusual cases, so they did not fit into my theme of "I wouldn't have believed it if I hadn't seen it with my own OR Eyes". This fact does not diminish the importance of having the recommended screening for colon cancer. Colon cancer is the # 3 cancer death here in the US. The guidelines pertaining to weight management and diet proposed in this book also pertain to colon cancer as well as colon cancer is highly associated with obesity and also smoking. It is of paramount importance to be screened for Colon cancer because of the untimely death due to this insidious disease and it is 99% preventable when precancerous polyps can be easily detected, and painlessly and easily removed via colonoscopy.

Always consult your **licensed** primary health professional for any questions regarding your health.

Writer's Biography

Kathy Volpe- Schaffer was born in Philadelphia, Pa. and was a long time resident of Philadelphia before moving to Southern New Jersey in 1981. She attended the Medical College of Pennsylvania Nursing School, which is now Drexel University and graduated in 1976. She obtained a BSN from Thomas Jefferson University in 1988 and later attended Rutgers's University in Camden, NJ and earned a Master's of Science degree in 1999 and likewise she earned her certification as a family nurse practitioner that same year. She also attended Rowan University in Glassboro, NJ, where she attained her NJ School Nursing certificate in 1996. She lives with her family in southern NJ where she has been a resident for the past 30 years.

Ten percent (10%) of the proceeds of this book will be donated to the National Multiple Sclerosis Society's (NMSS) College scholarship fund.